Pregnancy Q&A

Trish Booth

T0018836

 Meadowbrook Press

Distributed by Simon & Schuster
New York

Library of Congress Cataloging-in-Publication Data

Booth, Trish.
    Pregnancy Q & A: authoritative and reassuring answers to the questions on your mind / by
Trish Booth.
    p. cm.
    Includes index.
    ISBN 0-88166-476-6 (Meadowbrook) ISBN 0-684-02519-1 (Simon & Schuster)
    1. Pregnancy. 2. Childbirth. 3. Infants—Care. I. Title: Pregnancy Q and A. II. Title.

    RG556.B66 2004
    618.2—dc22

                                                                                    2004054660

Editorial Director: Christine Zuchora-Walske
Editor: Joseph Gredler
Proofreader: Angela Wiechmann
Production Manager: Paul Woods
Graphic Design Manager: Tamara Peterson
Indexer: Beverlee Day
Cover Photograph: © Rick Gomez

© 2004 by Trish Booth

All rights reserved. No part of this book may be reproduced or transmitted in any form or
by any means, electronic or mechanical, including photocopying, recording, or using any
information storage and retrieval system, without written permission from the publisher,
except in the case of brief quotations embodied in critical articles and reviews.

Although the author and publisher have made every effort to ensure that the information
in this book is accurate and current, only your care provider knows you and your medical
history well enough to make specific recommendations. The author, editors, reviewers, and
publisher disclaim any liability from the use of this book.

Published by Meadowbrook Press
5451 Smetana Drive
Minnetonka, MN 55343
www.meadowbrookpress.com

BOOK TRADE DISTRIBUTION by Simon and Schuster
a division of Simon and Schuster, Inc.
1230 Avenue of the Americas
New York, NY 10020

09 08 07 06 05 04   10 9 8 7 6 5 4 3 2 1

Printed in the United States of America

DEDICATION

To my husband, Jon,
and to Kathy, Jenna, Nathan,
Tyler, Jennifer, and Zachary,
who enrich my life as well
as my answers.

ACKNOWLEDGMENTS

When I stood in front of my first childbirth class in the fall of 1972, I hoped I had all the answers. Instead, I often found myself responding to questions by saying, "We'll talk about that next week." This gave me time to research and rehearse my answers. Every series of classes after that has been a learning experience for me. Thousands of expectant parents have prompted my search for answers while informing my responses. Some of my most profound learning experiences have come from listening to birth stories or witnessing births. To all those wonderful families who have shared their concerns, curiosities, and special moments of their lives, thank you.

My interactions and professional relationships with childbirth educators, midwives, and doulas in the United States, Canada, and South Africa have supported my growth as an educator and enhanced my listening as well as answering skills. I'd like to single out two educators in particular: Penny Simkin, for her ability to take research-based information and make it practical, and Linda Todd, for her insights that have lit my path into new topics, the most recent being post partum. To all my colleagues, thank you.

My interest in writing this book was sparked by answering my children's questions as they started their own families. I wanted to make sure my answers were factually accurate and emotionally appropriate. This was both challenging and gratifying. Kathy and Tyler, thank you.

This book is a reality because of the contributions of some important people. They are my reviewers Kim James, CD, CCE; Cheryl Kirchner, RN; Sue McDonald, CNM, MSN; Janet McGuigan, RN, CCE; and Sue Rio, RN, BSN, IBCLC, who generously shared their experience and wisdom; and my editor, Joseph Gredler, who gently asked questions until my answers were clear. Thank you all.

CONTENTS

INTRODUCTION

If you're already pregnant, congratulations! You're on a life-changing journey that will be filled with new experiences. As your baby grows, you'll be growing into parenthood. I wrote this book to help you navigate some of the wonders and challenges that lie ahead. If you're preparing for pregnancy, welcome. I hope reading this book helps you get ready for your journey.

Many of us live at a hectic pace and have little time for in-depth reading. Therefore, I've tried to make the information easily accessible by answering questions concisely. I've focused on questions women ask most often and those that are most important to address. I've also added practical tips and additional resources, such as books and websites, to allow you to pursue topics further. In addition, I've included information to help you talk with your care provider. Being able to effectively discuss your concerns with your provider is an important part of good prenatal care. Because your partner is also affected by your pregnancy, I've included tips to help the two of you talk about what's happening and plan for the future. I've even added some activities to help your partner interact with your developing baby.

Pregnant women have many questions about what's happening to their bodies. The response they often receive is, "Oh, that's normal." Yet, what's happening doesn't necessarily feel "normal." I've tried to answer these questions in a way that addresses women's wonderment and concerns.

Pregnancy is a special time and a healthy life event. That means you can build on a healthy lifestyle to have a healthy pregnancy. If you need to improve some of your choices, pregnancy may provide the motivation you need. Sustaining your changes will pay off for years to come.

During pregnancy you'll face decisions about tests and procedures related to your health and the health of your baby. You can use this book to get the basic information you need to talk with your care provider. Discussing options with your provider will enable you to make the best decisions for you and your baby.

Childbirth is timeless, but it's also influenced by the customs and procedures of your care provider and birth facility. Although each birth is unique, you can prepare for it by creating a birth plan. For example, consider how you want to cope with contractions, who your support people will be, and what you want those people to do. Some women practice coping skills ahead of time. Others don't. Reading the section on coping with labor and thinking about how you deal with physical stress and discomfort can help you decide what you want to do. Understanding the normal process of childbirth will make coping with it easier.

Giving birth brings you to the next trailhead: post partum. The work that immediately follows childbirth includes healing physically, establishing a relationship with your baby, renegotiating your other relationships, and adapting to parenthood. I've included practical tips on how to prepare for the first month after your baby is born. Although post partum lasts considerably longer, you'll be well on the path of parenthood by the end of the first month.

As you begin reading, you may want to focus on the questions that address what you're experiencing now. You can always revisit things you've experienced already and move ahead to what interests you. Feel free to skip over the questions that don't apply to your situation. I hope my answers help you assemble your resources and increase your enjoyment of this wondrous journey into parenthood.

Trish Booth

June 2004

SECTION ONE
Pregnancy

EARLY-PREGNANCY PLAN

Q I'M PREGNANT. NOW WHAT?

A A positive home pregnancy test means some decisions as well as celebration. Celebrate with your partner with a sparkling nonalcoholic
beverage and some favorite food. Then make an early pregnancy plan:
- If you haven't been taking a vitamin pill with folic acid, start now. You
  need at least 400 mcg (0.4 mg) of folic acid each day. (See page 14 for
  more on folic acid.)
- Don't drink any alcohol.
- Stop smoking.
- If you take medicines, call the care provider who prescribed them. Ask
  what to do now that you're pregnant.
- If you don't already know about your health insurance coverage, find out.
- Make an appointment with a prenatal care provider. (See pages 8–10 if
  you haven't chosen one.)
- Decide whom to tell and when. Although you may feel like spreading the
  news, many women tell only a few close friends and family members at first.
- Tell someone who can give you emotional support if you feel you're
  going to have to make a lot of changes.
- Start a savings account. Put your change in a jar or piggy bank. Add to it
  each night. Use the money to open a savings account for your baby or to
  buy something in honor of your baby's birth.
- Begin a pregnancy diary by recording how you felt when you found out
  you were pregnant.
- Write down five wishes for your baby.

TIMING THE PREGNANCY

Figuring the Due Date

Q MY HOME PREGNANCY TEST SAYS I'M PREGNANT.
HOW CAN I FIGURE OUT MY DUE DATE?

A It's relatively simple to calculate a due date. Take the date of the first
day of your last menstrual period and subtract three months. Then add
seven days. Finally, add a year.

You can also go online. Most pregnancy websites have a calendar that will figure out the date for you. Your prenatal care provider will compute the date at your first visit. If you can't remember the date of your last period or if you have irregular cycles, you may have to wait for an ultrasound to get a date.

On average, a pregnancy lasts 40 weeks (or 280 days) as figured from the date of the last period. However, your baby may be born between three weeks before and two weeks after your due date. Because fewer than 5 percent of babies are born on their due date, you may want to think in terms of a "due week."

Trimesters

Q WHY IS PREGNANCY DIVIDED INTO TRIMESTERS?

A Trimesters are a way to divide the nine months of pregnancy into thirds. That makes it easier to talk about the changes that occur with the woman and her developing baby. The first trimester actually starts before pregnancy because it's figured from the last menstrual period. It lasts through the 13th or 14th week. (There is some difference in how weeks are assigned.) The second trimester ends with the 26th or 27th week. The third trimester defines the remaining time until the baby is born, usually between the 38th and 40th week.

SIGNS OF PREGNANCY

Breast Changes

Q MY BREASTS ARE ALMOST TOO SORE TO TOUCH. WHAT'S HAPPENING?

A Your breasts are changing because of the hormones of pregnancy. In addition to getting larger, breasts get tender, especially around the nipple. These changes are often an early sign of pregnancy. Wearing a bra even at night may make you feel more comfortable. A stretchy sports bra is often a good choice. In addition, tell your partner about this increased sensitivity, as you may not want the usual amount of breast touching for a bit. The tenderness usually decreases after the first three months.

Q WHY DO MY BREASTS HAVE SO MANY RED AND BLUE LINES?

A Those colored lines are blood vessels. The blood supply to your breasts has increased as part of the changes that will create the ability to make milk and sustain breastfeeding. These blood vessels will be visible during pregnancy and while you're breastfeeding. They'll fade after you stop nursing.

Q THE AREA AROUND MY NIPPLE HAS GOTTEN DARKER AND HAS BUMPS. IS THAT NORMAL?

A Yes. The area around your nipple, called the areola, darkens during pregnancy. It's thought that this darkening makes it easier for the baby to see the nipple. After pregnancy, or when you stop breastfeeding, this coloration will fade. However, your areola will always be a little darker than it was before you got pregnant.

The little bumps on the areola are called Montgomery glands. They help lubricate the nipple area and keep it clean. Avoid squeezing or picking at these bumps because you don't want them to get infected. They'll slowly decrease in size after you give birth or are no longer nursing your baby. (See page 34 for other skin pigmentation changes.)

Q WILL I GET STRETCH MARKS ON MY BREASTS?

A You may. Some women get them more easily than others. When skin is stretched by rapid growth, the tissue just under the skin may separate, causing stretch marks. Lotion may help your skin feel more comfortable, but it won't prevent stretch marks. These will fade over time but won't completely disappear.

Bleeding or Spotting after a Missed Period

Q I'VE JUST FOUND OUT I'M PREGNANT, AND NOW I'M SPOTTING. SHOULD I BE WORRIED?

A Even though you stop having your periods when you're pregnant, you may have some bleeding or spotting early in pregnancy. A normal cause is implantation bleeding. This happens when the fertilized egg, which is now a ball of cells, burrows into the lining of the uterus. This occurs about 1 week to 10 days after conception. The amount of blood is usually slight. Some women bleed at the time they would have gotten their period. Contact your care provider to report your bleeding or spotting. That way it can be evaluated and you can ask whether to limit your activity. Be ready to describe the amount and color of the blood, how long you've been bleeding or spotting, and any pain or discomfort. Some care providers suggest that if the bleeding isn't heavy and there's no cramping or pain, no special precautions need to be taken. Women who have previously miscarried or who have had trouble getting pregnant may be told to rest until the bleeding stops. They also need to avoid activities that stimulate the uterus, like sex and nipple stimulation.

Morning Sickness

Q I HAVEN'T HAD ANY MORNING SICKNESS,
YET I KNOW I'M PREGNANT. IS THAT NORMAL?

A Morning sickness usually starts between the 4th and 6th weeks of pregnancy. Each woman experiences pregnancy differently. Not all pregnant women report morning sickness. Some only feel a bit queasy at times, most often when they have an empty stomach. You may be one of those women whose body has less difficulty adapting to the hormones of pregnancy.

Q I'M NAUSEATED MUCH OF THE DAY AND SOMETIMES VOMIT.
WILL THIS HURT MY BABY?

A Although it's called "morning" sickness, the nausea and vomiting of early pregnancy are not limited to the morning. Morning sickness is not a sign of a problem. Instead, it's a sign that your body is reacting to the hormones of pregnancy. Your occasional vomiting and limited food intake will not hurt your baby. Don't worry if you're not gaining weight. Eat what stays down. Most women feel a lot better when they get to the 12th week. Then they can start eating normally.

Ways to Cope with Morning Sickness

- Keep a little something in your stomach at all times.
  * Eat a little food many times during the day.
  * Low-fat foods and bland carbohydrates are often good choices when you feel queasy.
  * Avoid eating or drinking a lot at once.
  * Sip fluids throughout the day.
  * Eat a dry carbohydrate like crackers, rice cakes, toast, or some dry cereal before getting up in the morning.
  * Eat a small snack before going to bed.
  * If you get up during the night, nibble on something before going back to bed.
- Avoid anything that increases nausea.
  * Pregnancy brings an increased sense of smell, making women susceptible to nausea because of odors.
  * Many women find it difficult to handle or cook raw meat. If you do, have someone else cook that part of a meal.
- Try complementary therapies.
  * Ginger can be helpful in settling the stomach. Natural and whole-food stores sell ginger ales and ginger teas. You can also steep a piece of peeled fresh ginger about the size of a quarter in two cups of boiling water. Add honey or sugar and sip throughout the day.
  * You can buy acupressure wristbands (Sea-Bands) at most drugstores.
  * Ask your care provider about taking a vitamin B_6 supplement.

(See Hyperemesis Gravidarum on page 73.)

Frequent Urination

Q WHY DO I HAVE TO PEE ALL THE TIME?

A Your bladder and uterus are next to each other. At the start of pregnancy, your enlarging uterus presses on your bladder, which makes you feel the need to urinate. During the second trimester, there isn't as much pressure on your bladder because it moves up into your abdomen, where there's more room.

During the last few weeks of pregnancy, you'll again feel the need to urinate frequently because your baby and your very large uterus will be pressing on your bladder. (See pages 64–65 if you're having trouble with leaking urine.)

Q HOW CAN I REDUCE THE NUMBER OF TRIPS TO THE BATHROOM?

A It's never a good idea to try to hold your urine for a long period of time. Overfilling your bladder can cause tiny tears in the lining that can lead to an infection. Instead, focus on completely emptying your bladder. Leaning forward while urinating can help. Also, when you think you've finished urinating, stand up, then sit down and try again. Make sure to call your care provider if urination stings or burns. It could be a sign of a urinary tract infection.

If your ankles are swelling during the day, try putting your feet up above your heart for 15 minutes about an hour before going to bed. That will help get the fluid out of the cells and back into your bloodstream. Then you can get rid of that fluid by urinating before getting into bed.

You can also limit fluids after 6 PM. If you do this, however, you need to be drinking six to eight glasses (64 ounces) of fluid during the day. If you live in a very dry climate, check with your care provider about restricting your fluid during the evening hours.

Fatigue

Q I'M SO TIRED THAT SOMETIMES I CAN BARELY KEEP MY EYES OPEN. WILL I BE THIS TIRED THROUGHOUT MY WHOLE PREGNANCY?

A You're doing important and hard work growing a baby. In the first couple of months your body has to adjust to the hormonal changes of pregnancy. In addition, creating a baby and placenta makes your body expend a lot of energy, even if it doesn't feel like you're working hard. This leads to your feeling exhausted.

Fatigue may also be self-protective because being tired makes you reduce your activities. Most women get their energy back in the fourth month. If you don't, contact your care provider. You may be anemic. Anemia is usually treated with dietary changes and/or iron supplements. In the last month or so, you're likely to feel tired again. Carrying the weight of pregnancy and not getting as much sleep as usual will contribute to your fatigue. Until you feel more energetic, listen to your body and try to:

- Get as much sleep as you can at night. Go to bed as early as possible.
- Take a nap whenever you can. Even 15 minutes of rest can give you a lift. You may need to be creative in slipping a nap into your daytime routine.
- Reduce your commitments so you have time to take it easy.
- Eat well. Don't try to boost your energy with caffeine or high-sugar foods. They'll make you more tired when the immediate effect wears off.
- Try a little exercise. Walking, some gentle pregnancy exercises, or yoga may boost your energy level. (See pages 61–66 for more on exercise.)

CHOOSING A CARE PROVIDER

Q I'M CONCERNED ABOUT THE COST OF OBSTETRICAL CARE.

A Often an early concern is the cost of care. If you have health insurance, confirm your coverage directly with your insurance carrier. The company can provide the details of your policy as well as a list of approved providers.

If you don't have insurance, you may be eligible for state or federally funded healthcare. Go online or contact your local or state health department for program details.

You can also call prospective providers to determine if they have a sliding fee scale or payment plan. Community clinics are often a cost-effective option.

Q ARE THERE DIFFERENT KINDS OF CARE PROVIDERS?

A Most obstetrical care providers are either physicians or midwives. An obstetrician (OB) is a physician who specializes in pregnancy and birth. Many obstetricians are also gynecologists. You may have already been seeing this person for your Pap tests and other gynecological care. OBs are specialists; they can diagnose and treat complications of childbirth as well as take care of normal pregnancies. Some obstetricians specialize in high-risk pregnancies.

A family physician is a physician who has received training in pregnancy and birth but is not a specialist. In addition to providing maternity care, this physician can care for your baby after birth. You may have already been seeing this person for your general healthcare. Family physicians usually refer to an obstetrician if there are pregnancy or birth complications.

A certified nurse midwife (CNM) is a nurse who has received additional training in normal pregnancy and birth. Many CNMs also provide basic gynecological care. Midwives focus on maintaining a healthy pregnancy and schedule visits that allow time for questions. They may work as part of a clinic or private practice, or on their own with physician backup. If there's a complication, they refer to an obstetrician.

There are also midwives who are not trained as nurses. Their training and experience varies. Depending on where you live, there may be midwives licensed by the state or certified by an organization. These midwives usually attend home births or work in birth centers. For more information visit the American College of Nurse-Midwives website at www.acnm.org.

Tips on Finding an Obstetrical Care Provider

It's important that you feel comfortable with your obstetrical care provider. Consider the following:

- How active do you want to be in the decision making? Do you want to take an active role, or would you prefer to rely on the provider's recommendation without having to explore the issue?
- Do you want specific things during your labor and birth? Are you planning on using professional labor support such as a doula? Do you have strong preferences related to procedures or pain control?
- Do you prefer to get care from a man or woman? Does your religion or culture affect your choice? Physicians can be either men or women. Most midwives are women.
- Does the type of practice matter? Many physicians and midwives practice as part of a group. That means that the members of the practice share an on-call schedule. The person who assists your birth will be the person on-call for that day (or night). You may see the other members of the practice during your scheduled prenatal visits.

  Some providers have a solo practice and attempt to be at the births of all their patients. They have another provider cover for them when they can't make a birth. You may or may not meet that provider beforehand. You may also have to wait or reschedule a prenatal visit if the provider is assisting at a birth.
- Does the location of the office or clinic matter? If your work is a considerable distance from your home, you may want to see a provider nearer your work to minimize time away from your job.

Q WHAT'S A GOOD WAY TO FIND A CARE PROVIDER?

A First, consider the questions on page 9. Then, when you have some idea of your preferences:

- Ask your general healthcare provider for recommendations.
- Ask friends and colleagues for recommendations. Listen carefully to *why* the person liked the provider. Do you share those concerns and priorities?
- If you're interested in using a specific hospital or birth center, call that facility to get a list of providers who practice there.
- Ask a local independent childbirth education group or a hospital's child-birth education coordinator for the names of providers who refer families to their classes.

After you have an idea of what you're looking for in a provider, call the office or clinic of your top choices to get further information. If you cannot decide between providers, schedule an informational appointment to speak to a prospective provider in person.

CHOOSING A BIRTH SITE

Q WHAT'S THE DIFFERENCE BETWEEN A BIRTHING ROOM AND A BIRTH CENTER?

A A birth center is usually a freestanding center that provides labor, birth, and immediate postpartum services. These centers provide care for women who are planning a vaginal birth. Many also provide prenatal care. A woman goes to the birth center when she's in labor and stays for a period of time after giving birth, usually less than a day. Family members and others of the woman's choosing are welcome. Birth centers offer a homelike setting and a minimum of medical interventions. If the woman or her baby requires more intensive care, she's transported to a nearby hospital. For more information about birth centers visit www.birthcenters.org.

A birthing room is a room in a hospital in which a woman labors and gives birth. Usually family members and others who are providing support can be with her. Most procedures are done in this room. In some hospitals the woman spends her whole hospital stay in this room. In other facilities she moves to a postpartum room a few hours after giving birth. If the woman needs a cesarean, she's taken to an operating suite.

Q WHAT IF I WANT A HOME BIRTH?

A Some women having normal, healthy pregnancies choose to give birth at home. Although home birth has a good safety record, it may be difficult to find a care provider. Most physicians and many certified nurse midwives will not attend a home birth. You may need to find a birth attendant or certified midwife (a midwife who is not a nurse). She will provide prenatal care and education as well as attend the birth. She will also advise you about the supplies you'll need to have on hand. In addition, she'll explain under what conditions she transports her clients to the hospital. If an expectant woman has a health condition or a complicated pregnancy, it's safer for her to give birth in a hospital.

PRENATAL VISITS

Q WHAT CAN I EXPECT AT MY FIRST PRENATAL VISIT?

A Your first visit is likely to be your longest. In addition to confirming the pregnancy and estimating your due date, your care provider will check your general health. This will include a physical exam, a review of your health history, and a blood drawing for a series of tests. If you're a new patient and haven't received forms to fill out beforehand, come prepared with dates of past pregnancies, illnesses, injuries, and surgeries; information about your family's health, especially genetic problems; and medicines you're taking. Make sure to bring all your health insurance information.

There will also be time to ask questions. Write them down ahead of time because it's easy to forget them in the rush of all that's being done.

Q WILL THE OTHER VISITS BE LIKE THE FIRST ONE?

A The remaining visits are usually much shorter. They're designed to monitor your health and your baby's growth. They involve checking a urine sample, checking your weight and blood pressure, measuring the growth of your uterus, and (starting in the third month) listening to your baby's heart. Throughout your pregnancy your provider will order specific tests and usually an ultrasound or two. Even though the visits are shorter, come prepared to ask whatever questions you have.

Q HOW FREQUENTLY ARE PRENATAL VISITS SCHEDULED?

A The most common pattern is one visit per month until the seventh month, then every two weeks until the last month. At that point they're weekly until you give birth. You'll be seen more frequently if there's a need to monitor or treat a problem.

Q I SEEM TO HAVE MORE QUESTIONS THAN MY PROVIDER HAS TIME FOR. WHAT CAN I DO ABOUT THIS?

A The pace of a visit can leave little time for in-depth conversation. However, it's important that your questions get answered. Do you have general questions about pregnancy and birth, or are they specific to you? The time is best spent on questions that relate specifically to your pregnancy. You may be able to get many of your general questions answered by reading books such as *Pregnancy, Childbirth, and the Newborn* (by Simkin, Whalley, and Keppler), by taking an early-pregnancy or prenatal class, by talking to a nurse or educator in the practice, or by visiting websites such as the Cleveland Clinic Health Information Center (www.clevelandclinic.org/health; click on "Pregnancy" then "Written Materials").

Write down your questions and ask your most pressing ones first. In addition, explain to your provider that you have unanswered questions. Ask to schedule a phone consultation or an additional visit, if necessary. Giving your provider a written list of questions might also help.

Q SHOULD MY PARTNER COME TO MY PRENATAL VISITS?

A That's something you and your partner should talk about. Going to the prenatal visits may help your partner feel more involved in the pregnancy. The visits also give your partner a chance to get his or her questions answered. In addition, it's easier to remember what the care provider said when two people are listening. Your partner can even take notes. Most partners like going to an ultrasound appointment because they can "see" the baby. To schedule a visit that minimizes time away from work:

• Ask if the office or clinic has evening or Saturday appointments.
• Ask for the first morning appointment because you're less likely to have to wait.

- The last afternoon appointment may start late but may be convenient if you don't have to return to work.

If your partner can't make the visits:
- Talk with your partner beforehand about questions and concerns.
- Write down your partner's questions. That way you can pull out the list and make sure the questions get answered.

CALLING YOUR CARE PROVIDER

Q I RECENTLY CALLED MY DOCTOR, AND THE CONVERSATION WAS VERY FRUSTRATING FOR BOTH OF US. HOW CAN I GET THE ATTENTION I NEED BETWEEN SCHEDULED OFFICE VISITS?

A It's important to call your care provider's office when you're ill or concerned about your or your baby's health. (See page 73 for warning signs that indicate you should contact your provider.) Here are some things you can do to help your provider help you:
- Try to call during office hours. That way your provider can look at your chart and give you a more complete answer.
- Leave a telephone number where your provider can reach you, even if your call is returned after the office closes.
- Have a pen and paper ready to write down instructions.
- Before you call, write down important information including:
  * Your due date or the number of weeks you're pregnant;
  * When you were last seen in the office, and whether it was a routine visit;
  * Exactly what you're concerned about.
  * If you're feeling ill:
    - Your symptoms, when they started, and how they've progressed;
    - Your temperature;
    - Whether you've been exposed to anything;
    - If this is a follow-up call, what you've been previously told to do.
- Have the name and phone number of your pharmacy available.

HEALTHY EATING

Nutrition

Q WHY IS IT IMPORTANT THAT I GET ENOUGH FOLIC ACID WHILE I'M PREGNANT?

A Folic acid (folate) is a B vitamin that's important to your baby's development. A folic-acid deficiency has been linked with birth defects of the brain and spinal cord as well as cleft lip and cleft palate. The most important time to be taking folic acid is from your last menstrual period through the first five weeks of pregnancy. It's now recommended that women of childbearing age get at least 4oo mcg (0.4 mg) of folic acid each day. Foods rich in folate include whole grains and leafy green vegetables. Most daily vitamin tablets, including prenatal vitamins, contain the recommended dose. Because folic acid is important to everyone's health, flour, bread, and some cereals made in the United States are now fortified with folic acid.

Tips for Having a Healthy Pregnancy

- Get prenatal care.
- Eat a variety of healthy foods.
- Exercise.
- Maintain a normal weight.
- Avoid alcohol.
- Avoid smoking and tobacco smoke.
- Avoid drugs and over-the-counter medicines unless prescribed by your care provider.

Q ARE OTHER VITAMINS IMPORTANT DURING PREGNANCY?

A Vitamins are important for the growth of your baby and for the absorption of nutrients. They help keep your body working well. Your daily prenatal vitamin ensures that you're getting all that you need, but it's best to get a majority of your vitamins from food sources. Eat a variety of fruits and vegetables each day, at least five servings.
- Vitamin C is important for tissue formation and the absorption of iron. Citrus fruit, strawberries, raspberries, papaya, tomatoes, and peppers are good sources. Choose at least two servings. (See page 17 for more on servings.) Eat these foods fresh and uncooked because light, heat, and air destroy vitamin C.

- Eat at least one serving of a leafy green vegetable and one serving of a yellow or orange fruit or vegetable. These provide a variety of important vitamins including vitamin A and the B vitamins. Some also contain vitamin C. Leafy green vegetables include spinach, broccoli, kale, and beet or collard greens. Look at the inside of the fruit or vegetable to determine its color. Yellow or orange produce includes carrots, winter squash, sweet potatoes, yams, mangoes, and cantaloupe.
- Have at least one serving of another vegetable or fruit such as green beans, asparagus, summer squash, bananas, apples, and blueberries. They provide additional vitamins and minerals as well as antioxidants that keep the body healthy.
- Aim to have only one fruit or vegetable serving in the form of juice. Fruit juices in particular can add many calories. Eating the actual fruit or vegetable provides dietary fiber that drinking juice doesn't.
- The body does not store water-soluble vitamins like C and the B complex. This means you need to eat foods rich in these vitamins each day.
- Fat-soluble vitamins are stored in body fat. This means that an excess amount of the vitamin can be toxic. Vitamin A is of concern because it can cause birth defects at high doses. Getting a lot of vitamins from the foods you eat is not a concern if you eat a varied diet. Avoid taking megadoses of vitamins.

Q I KNOW PREGNANT WOMEN NEED A LOT OF CALCIUM. WHY?

A Calcium is a mineral that's needed to build bones and teeth. When you increase the amount of calcium in your diet, you give your body the calcium it needs for your developing baby. If you don't get enough of it, your body will start to take it from your bones. Your muscles also use calcium. When you don't get enough calcium, you may have muscle cramps. You need 1200 grams of calcium each day, the amount found in four glasses (32 ounces) of milk.

Q I DON'T LIKE THE TASTE OF MILK. HOW ELSE CAN I GET THE CALCIUM I NEED?

A You can flavor milk, eat other dairy products, and use other sources of calcium. If you vary your calcium sources, it might not feel like such a chore to get the 1200 grams you need. Here are some options to try:
- Make a fruit smoothie with milk or yogurt.
- Steam or heat milk, and add a flavoring.
- Dip vegetables in plain yogurt seasoned with dill.
- Dip fruits in yogurt sweetened with honey or brown sugar.

- Add grated low-fat cheese to pasta dishes and casseroles.
- Treat yourself to frozen yogurt or low-fat ice cream.
- Drink fruit juice or soymilk fortified with calcium.
- Add calcium-fortified tofu, cooked dried beans, and peas to salads and rice dishes.
- Snack on calcium-fortified ready-to-eat cereals like Total.
- Take a calcium supplement. To ensure maximum absorption of calcium, when you take the supplement also eat a food containing vitamin D or choose a supplement that contains vitamin D.

Q I KNOW YOU NEED IRON FOR MAKING RED BLOOD CELLS. HOW CAN I GET THE IRON I NEED EACH DAY?

A Your body needs significantly more iron when you're pregnant. You have to create additional red blood cells in order to carry the oxygen you and your baby need. In addition, your developing baby needs iron to build red blood cells. You'll be getting some iron from the meat you eat as well as from fruits, vegetables, and grains. Because it's difficult to get all the iron you need from food, most care providers suggest an iron supplement. The dosage depends on whether you had low iron stores or were iron deficient before getting pregnant. Eating foods rich in vitamin C helps increase iron absorption. Iron supplements can cause constipation and intestinal distress. Talk with your care provider about the best iron supplement for you.

Q HOW MUCH PROTEIN DO I NEED NOW THAT I'M PREGNANT?

A You need 60–75 grams of protein a day. You can get this in two to three servings of meat, fish, or eggs. (See page 17.) Dairy products and grains also provide protein, but in lesser amounts. Most Americans eat more than enough protein each day.

Q I'M A VEGETARIAN. DO I HAVE TO WORRY ABOUT MY PROTEIN INTAKE?

A If you eat eggs and milk, you can easily get the protein you need. If you're a vegan, you can get enough protein by eating six to eight servings of plant-based proteins. Make sure to include a variety of whole grains, legumes, and nuts. If you're not certain that you're getting enough protein, ask your care provider for a referral to a nutritionist.

Q ARE WHOLE GRAINS THAT DIFFERENT FROM AN ENRICHED PRODUCT?

A Whole grains, as the name implies, have all of the grain. They're more nutritious than refined grains because the refining process strips away most of the nutrients. Even when nutrients are added back, some are still left out. Whole grains also have more fiber in addition to a richer supply of vitamins, minerals, and protein. If you're not used to the taste and texture of whole grains, start by mixing white and brown rice or adding whole-grain flour to white.

Helpful Serving Sizes

- Grains: 1 slice of bread; 1 tortilla; ½ cup cooked pasta or rice; 1 ounce dry cereal
- Vegetables: 1 cup raw (for leafy vegetables); ½ cup raw or cooked (for others)
- Fruits: 1 medium (fits in the palm of your hand); ½ cup diced; ¾ cup juice
- Milk and dairy products: 1 cup milk or yogurt; 1-inch cube of hard cheese
- Meat and eggs: 2–3 ounces of meat or poultry (about the size of a deck of cards); 2–3 eggs
- Vegetable protein: ½ cup cooked dried beans or 1½ tablespoons of peanut butter are equal to 1 ounce of meat

Q WHAT DO YOU MEAN WHEN YOU REFER TO "SERVINGS"?

A Nutritional information is based on a standardized amount called a serving. It's not the same as a portion or helping. Many serving sizes are a lot smaller than most people usually serve. This can be helpful when it leads to getting more of the "good." For example, the fluid recommendation is eight to ten glasses a day based on a one-cup (eight-ounce) glass. Many glasses hold 12 ounces, meaning you'd need to fill your glass fewer times.

It can also mean that you're getting more of a less healthful thing. When estimating the amount of caffeine in a cup of coffee, that cup is only 8 ounces. If you're drinking coffee out of a mug, you may be drinking several cups at a time. Once you know what a serving size is, you don't have to measure everything you eat. You can look at a portion and estimate if it's more or less than a serving.

Weight Gain

Q HOW MUCH WEIGHT AM I SUPPOSED TO GAIN?

A The recommended weight gain depends on several factors that are unique to each woman. These include her age, her weight before pregnancy, and the number of babies she's carrying. A common recommendation is that women of normal weight gain between 25 and 35 pounds. A teenager may be asked to gain around 35 pounds because she's still growing. A woman who's underweight might also be asked to gain around 35 pounds. A woman who's significantly overweight can usually safely limit weight gain to about 20 pounds. However, it's important that she gain at least 15 pounds in order to get the nutrition she and her baby need. Pregnancy is not the time to try to lose weight. Women who are carrying more than one baby need to gain more than 35 pounds. However, they don't need to gain twice the usual recommendation. Your care provider will help you set a goal for your pregnancy weight gain.

Q WHO DETERMINES WHAT NORMAL WEIGHT IS?

A Most care providers use a body mass index (BMI) table to determine a person's weight status. You can figure out your BMI by using this formula:

$$\frac{\text{Your weight in pounds}}{\text{Your height in inches squared}} \times 703 = \text{BMI}$$

A person with a BMI below 18.5 is considered underweight. A normal BMI is between 18.5 and 24.9. A person with a BMI between 25 and 29.9 is considered overweight. A person with a BMI above 30 is considered obese by international standards. You can also determine your BMI online by visiting www.aafp.org/x24180.xml or www.cdc.gov/nccdphp/dnpa/bmi.

Q WHERE DOES THE PREGNANCY WEIGHT GO?

A The weight gain comes from changes in your body, the systems that support your baby, and your baby's weight. These add up to about 23 pounds. Your body also needs to store some fat to make sure you have enough energy to meet your new baby's demands. If there's only one baby, weight gain above 30 pounds consists mostly of stored fat.

Q WHAT DOES THIS WEIGHT GAIN MEAN IN TERMS OF MY DAILY EATING HABITS?

A It takes about 300 extra calories a day to grow a baby. That's the number of calories in a peanut-butter sandwich or 8 ounces of low-fat yogurt and an apple. As you can see, that really isn't a lot of extra food. That's why it's helpful to focus on eating well. (See pages 14–17 for more on healthy eating.)

Approximate Distribution of a Thirty-Pound Weight Gain at the End of Pregnancy

Breast changes	1–2 pounds
Increased blood volume	3–4 pounds
Increased fluid in body tissues	3–4 pounds
Larger uterus	2 pounds
Amniotic fluid	2 pounds
Placenta	1½ pounds
Baby	7½ pounds
Fat stores	7–10 pounds

Q HOW IMPORTANT IS IT TO GAIN THE RECOMMENDED AMOUNT OF WEIGHT?

A Weight gain recommendations are just that, recommendations. If you gain less than the recommended amount, you may not be able to get all the nutrients you and your baby need. This can affect your baby's growth and development. Gaining more than the recommended weight may put you at increased risk for medical problems and can increase pregnancy discomforts. It also means you'll have more weight to lose after your baby is born. Although some women who gain a lot of weight during pregnancy lose the weight gradually over the next year, other women find it difficult to get back to their prepregnancy weight. Because the most important issue is getting the nutrients you and your baby need, it's best to focus on eating healthy foods throughout pregnancy rather than fixating on weight gain.

Q DOES IT MATTER HOW QUICKLY I GAIN WEIGHT?

A It's best to gain weight steadily over the course of your pregnancy, which is in keeping with your baby's needs. During the first three months, it's suggested that you gain around a pound a month. Your developing baby is very small, and you don't need a lot of extra nutrition at this time. Some women lose a little weight due to nausea and vomiting, but this doesn't harm the baby. Women who are underweight are often asked to gain more in the first trimester so they're closer to their ideal weight before the baby makes greater nutritional demands.

After the first trimester, most care providers suggest that expectant mothers gain about a pound a week. In reality, weight isn't usually gained at this ideal rate. Some weeks it's a little more; others a little less. The goal is to gain weight as steadily as you can so your baby gets a continuous supply of nutrients for optimal growth and development.

Q I GAINED A LOT OF WEIGHT IN THE FIRST TRIMESTER. NOW WHAT DO I DO?

A The best thing to do is look at what you're eating each day and make sure you're making healthy choices. You can slow weight gain by reducing fat and sugar intake. Snack on fruits and vegetables instead of chips and cookies. Drink low-fat or skim milk instead of whole milk. Drink water instead of soda, fruit-flavored drinks, or fruit juice. If you're having trouble identifying changes you need to make, ask your care provider for a referral to a nutritionist.

Q I'M FINDING IT VERY DIFFICULT TO EAT ENOUGH FOOD TO GAIN THE WEIGHT I'M SUPPOSED TO.

A Women who are very thin before getting pregnant may find it difficult to eat enough food each day. That means they need to make sure everything they eat is nutrient rich. Choose foods that satisfy at least two nutrient requirements, such as milk or yogurt for calcium and protein, dark vegetables for multiple vitamins, and whole grains for fiber, vitamins, and minerals. Drink 100 percent fruit juices and smoothies as part of your daily fluids. Eliminate all junk food, and instead snack on nuts, whole-grain crackers, and cheese. Try eating five or six smaller meals each day rather than three large ones.

Q I EAT OUT A LOT. HOW CAN I KEEP FROM GAINING MORE WEIGHT THAN I SHOULD?

A Eating at restaurants, whether fast-food or fancy, can be a challenge to healthy eating. The two biggest challenges are serving size and the higher fat and sugar content of the food. To reduce the amount of food you eat:
• Try to avoid viewing the restaurant meal as a splurge.

- Consider the restaurant meal your biggest meal of the day. Size your other meals accordingly.
- Share an entrée and order a side salad if you're still hungry.
- Order a small salad and appetizer rather than a regular meal.
- Order the smallest size possible. Or ask if you can have a half order or an appetizer portion. Avoid super sizing.
- Ask for a take-home carton when your meal is served. Immediately put half the food into the container to eat at another meal.

To minimize excess calories:
- Look for "heart-healthy" and "low-fat" designations on the menu.
- Ask for dressings or gravy on the side.
- Order burgers and sandwiches without mayonnaise and special sauces.
- Substitute mustard for fatty spreads and yogurt for sour cream.
- Order meat, poultry, or fish stir-fried, broiled, or grilled. Avoid battered and fried foods.
- Order a salad rather than a burger.
- Drink a glass of water during the meal.
- Share a dessert if you're having one.

FOOD SAFETY

Fish

Q WITH ALL THE NEWS ABOUT MERCURY, HOW SAFE IS IT TO EAT FISH?

A Because mercury can cause brain damage in babies, pregnant and nursing women have been warned to avoid eating large saltwater fish that are most likely to contain mercury. Until recently, this warning applied to four types of fish: shark, king mackerel, swordfish, and tilefish. Now there's concern about the amount of mercury in tuna.

Fish are a good source of protein and the omega-3 fatty acids that promote nervous system development. They are a healthful food choice, even for pregnant women. It seems reasonable to have up to four three-ounce servings a week coming from a variety of fish and shellfish. When choosing canned tuna, light tuna is better than albacore because it's a smaller fish.

Q WHAT ABOUT PCBs IN SALMON?

A PCBs, industrial pollutants known to cause cancer, have been found in farm-raised salmon. This contamination comes from the food these salmon are fed. Wild salmon contain considerably less PCBs. Some salmon suppliers have begun testing their fish for PCBs and providing information to help buyers choose products.

Q DO I NEED TO WORRY ABOUT EATING LOCAL FRESHWATER FISH?

A Sometimes local fish can be contaminated with pesticides or industrial chemicals. It's best to contact your local health department to find out what's recommended.

Food Safety Tips

- Wash your hands thoroughly before handling food.
- Rinse all produce thoroughly under running water.
- Check the origin of produce. Currently, foreign-grown produce is inspected less than US-grown. If the produce can easily become contaminated with sewage while it's being grown, peel or cook it before eating. The highest risk comes from fruits and vegetables that grow lying on the ground, such as cantaloupe and zucchini.
- Consider buying organic produce to reduce exposure to pesticides.
- Buy only pasteurized dairy products and fruit juices.
- Refrigerate foods as needed.
  * Check the label to see if the food needs to be refrigerated after opening.
  * Don't leave prepared food out for more than two hours. Refrigerate or freeze leftovers as soon as possible.
- Thaw foods in the refrigerator or microwave, not on the counter.
- Do not eat raw eggs or seafood.
- Handle raw meat carefully.
  * Keep it away from other foods.
  * Wash utensils and cutting boards in hot soapy water after they've come in contact with raw meat.
  * Dedicate a nonporous cutting board for meat preparation.
- Cook all meats thoroughly. Get an instant-read thermometer so you can determine the internal temperature.

Listeriosis

Q I'VE HEARD YOUR BABY CAN GET VERY SICK OR DIE IF YOU GET AN ILLNESS FROM EATING SOFT CHEESE. WHAT CAN I DO TO AVOID THIS?

A Listeriosis is a rare food-borne illness that starts with flu-like symptoms or intestinal upset. It can result in premature labor, miscarriage, or stillbirth when a woman is pregnant. Babies born with the disease are very ill.

The best way to prevent listeriosis is to avoid risky foods. The listeria bacteria are most commonly found in unpasteurized milk and milk products, especially soft cheeses such as feta and Brie, deli meats (hot dogs, bologna, and liverwurst), and liver pâtés. Check labels to make sure milk products are pasteurized. Cook hot dogs and deli meats before eating them. It may be safest to avoid pâtés while you're pregnant. Listeria can also be found in precooked take-home meals such as chicken or seafood, so reheat them thoroughly.

DRUGS

Alcohol

Q WHY ARE PREGNANT WOMEN TOLD NOT TO DRINK ALCOHOL?

A Drinking alcohol throughout pregnancy increases the risk of miscarriage, stillbirth, prematurity, and low birth weight. It also causes neurological problems and mental retardation. Scientists are discovering that even small amounts of alcohol taken consistently can have negative effects for the baby. In the second trimester, alcohol interferes with brain development. In the third trimester, it kills existing brain cells and interrupts nervous system development. The harm that is done can have lifelong consequences. Because no one knows what a safe amount is, it's best to avoid alcohol use.

Q WHAT IS FETAL ALCOHOL SYNDROME?

A Some mothers who drink heavily throughout pregnancy have babies who are born with a collection of birth defects known as fetal alcohol syndrome (FAS). These include growth retardation, facial deformities, and central nervous system damage. FAS children have learning disabilities, poor coordination, social and behavioral problems, and poor judgment. They may also have other health problems.

Q IF A BABY DOESN'T HAVE FAS,
DOES THAT MEAN THE ALCOHOL DIDN'T CAUSE ANY DAMAGE?

A Unfortunately, no. Many babies who are consistently exposed to alcohol while in the womb show some effects. These include developmental delays, coordination problems, and attention deficits. The problem may be subtle or quite striking. It depends on the mother's drinking pattern.

Q WHICH IS WORSE, HAVING ONE DRINK A DAY FOR FIVE DAYS OR HAVING FIVE DRINKS ON ONE DAY AND NOT DRINKING ON THE OTHER FOUR?

A Binge drinking (drinking a lot of alcohol at one time) is worse. The alcohol in the mother's blood crosses the placenta and goes into the baby's blood. The high level of alcohol damages the baby's brain.

Q I HAD A LOT TO DRINK ON THE NIGHT I GOT PREGNANT.
DID THAT HARM MY BABY?

A The first two weeks of pregnancy, from conception until the ball of cells burrows into the lining of the uterus, is a protected time. A baby is not affected by the mother's drinking. You did not harm your baby by drinking on that night.

Q IS WINE OR BEER SAFER THAN DISTILLED SPIRITS LIKE VODKA AND WHISKEY?

A No. It's the alcohol, not the source of the alcohol, that causes the problem. A can or bottle of beer, a glass of wine, and a shot of liquor each contain about the same amount of alcohol.

Smoking

Q HOW IMPORTANT IS IT TO QUIT SMOKING WHEN YOU'RE PREGNANT?

A Very. Smoking affects circulation and exposes both the mother and the baby to harmful chemicals. Every time a pregnant woman smokes, her baby gets less oxygen. The nicotine in the cigarette smoke reduces blood flow to the placenta. At the same time, the carbon monoxide decreases the amount of oxygen the blood can carry. In addition, there are toxic chemicals that can hurt a developing baby. Smoking also increases the risk of pregnancy complications, miscarriage, and stillbirth.

Babies born to mothers who smoked during pregnancy are smaller than babies born to non-smokers. They're also more likely to be born too early and have immediate health problems. During infancy they get more illnesses, are hospitalized more, and are more likely to die of sudden infant death syndrome (SIDS). Tobacco smoke also harms brain development. As a result, these babies are more likely to have learning and behavioral problems later in life.

Ways to Quit Smoking

- Begin a program to stop smoking. The American Lung Association has a program for pregnant women. Go online and visit www.lungusa.org/tobacco/ffs_baby.html.
- Ask your care provider for a referral to a local smoking cessation program.
- If you need more help, consider adding hypnosis or acupuncture.
- Talk with your care provider about prescription aids to help you stop smoking.
- It's never too late to quit. If you can't quit, at least cut back. The damage done by smoking increases with the number of cigarettes you smoke. Every cigarette you don't smoke is a gift to your baby.

Q I'VE STOPPED SMOKING BUT MY PARTNER STILL SMOKES. WHAT SHOULD I DO?

A Secondhand smoke has the same harmful effects on a developing baby as direct smoking. Keep as many places in your life as smoke-free as possible:

- Ask your partner not to smoke around you.
- Make the car a smoke-free zone.
- Have your partner smoke outside or in the garage. If that's not possible, limit smoking to one well-ventilated room. Stay out of that room as much as possible.
- When you go out, consider going to places where smoking is prohibited.
- Support your partner's efforts to reduce or quit smoking. You know firsthand how hard it can be to stop smoking.

Caffeine

Q DO I HAVE TO GIVE UP DRINKING COFFEE?

A Although you don't have to give up coffee, it's probably best to limit your daily caffeine intake. Caffeine is a stimulant that narrows blood vessels. This affects your baby's oxygen and nutrient supply. In addition, caffeine is a diuretic that causes your body to get rid of fluid and some calcium. Most care providers suggest consuming less than 300 mg a day, so one to two cups is fine. The amount of caffeine in coffee varies considerably depending on the type of bean, roast, and preparation. Instant coffee has the least amount.

If you don't want to give up drinking coffee, consider switching to decaf after the first cup, or make half-caf by creating a blend of regular and decaffeinated beans.

Q DO I HAVE TO WORRY ABOUT CAFFEINE EVEN THOUGH I DON'T DRINK COFFEE?

A Other beverages, chocolate, and some medicines contain caffeine. An eight-ounce cup of black tea contains about 50 mg. A cup of green tea has about 30 mg. A twelve-ounce can of cola or other caffeinated soft drink has about 50 mg. A chocolate bar usually has about 30 mg.

If you want to lower your caffeine consumption, drink decaffeinated black or green tea. Herbal teas usually don't contain caffeine. However, some herbs should be avoided in pregnancy. Check with your care provider about the safety of the teas you like.

There are caffeine-free soft drinks. However, pregnancy is a good time to switch to water or more healthful beverages. Consider drinking flavored sparkling water or mixing a small amount of pure fruit juice with sparkling or noncarbonated water.

Medicines

Q WHAT OVER-THE-COUNTER DRUGS ARE SAFE TO TAKE DURING PREGNANCY?

A It's best not to take any medicines without talking to your care provider first. Then take as little as you can. Many providers recommend acetaminophen (Tylenol) for pain. After the first trimester, pseudoephedrine

(Sudafed) is often used as a decongestant. Tums and Maalox are often recommended antacids for relief of heartburn. Providers, however, usually have their own preferences for relief of pregnancy-related problems.

Q WHAT ABOUT HERBS AND NATURAL REMEDIES?

A Herbs and natural remedies can affect a developing baby. Their active ingredients are drugs. Talk with your care provider about the herbs and remedies you take or plan to take. If you need immediate information about the effect of an herb, call the American Association of Poison Control Centers at 800-222-1222. Herbal products are not regulated for purity or strength the way medicines are. It's best to look for suppliers who test their products to maintain a standard.

Q ARE PRESCRIPTION MEDICINES SAFE TO TAKE DURING PREGNANCY?

A Although many prescription drugs can be safe to take during pregnancy, there are a few that can affect the way a baby develops. Make sure the care provider who is prescribing your medicine knows that you're pregnant. Don't discontinue a prescribed drug on your own. If you have concerns about a medication you're taking, contact your care provider. In addition, bring a list of all medicines you're taking to your first prenatal visit.

Recreational Drugs

Q DOES SMOKING MARIJUANA WHEN YOU'RE PREGNANT HURT THE BABY?

A It's not considered safe to smoke marijuana. Long-term studies of children who were exposed to marijuana in the womb show effects on brain development. This includes behavioral problems, such as poor impulse control, and a decreased ability to solve complex problems.

Q ARE THERE ANY SAFE RECREATIONAL DRUGS?

A Recreational (street) drugs and abused prescription drugs pose a number of risks. Although they're not likely to cause birth defects, they do affect development. A few, like crack and cocaine, endanger the baby's blood and oxygen supply. They can also cause a baby to be born too early. Some drugs affect brain development or result in low birth weight. Others, like hallucinogens, harm the mother's ability to make good decisions. These risks may be compounded when the drugs are used in combination with each other or with alcohol. (See pages 23–24 for more on alcohol use.) If a mother is addicted to a drug, her baby will go through withdrawal symptoms after birth. Babies who are born with drugs in their systems are often jittery and irritable, harder to calm, and cry a lot. This is hard on both the mother and the baby. If you find you cannot stop using drugs, tell your care provider. There are recovery programs designed for pregnant women.

ENVIRONMENTAL CONCERNS

Toxoplasmosis

Q WHAT DO I HAVE TO DO REGARDING MY CAT AND TOXOPLASMOSIS?

A Toxoplasmosis is an illness that's spread in the feces of infected cats. The illness is usually not serious in adults. It can, however, cause severe problems in a developing baby, especially during the first trimester. If you've had your cat for a while and the cat goes outdoors, you may already be immune. There's a blood test to determine immunity. It's usually done prior to pregnancy or to verify a suspected active illness. If you're not sure you're immune, take precautions to avoid coming in contact with the parasite. Let someone else clean the litter box, and wash your hands thoroughly if you come in contact with cat feces. Because you can get toxoplasmosis other ways, see the precautions below.

Q DO I HAVE TO WORRY ABOUT TOXOPLASMOSIS EVEN THOUGH I DON'T HAVE A CAT?

A Yes, you can still become exposed to the *Toxoplasma gondii* parasite through garden soil or a sandbox containing cat feces. Wear gloves when you garden and wash your hands when you're finished. Keep sandboxes covered when not in use.

You can also get toxoplasmosis from food. The soil clinging to vegetables may have been contaminated with the parasite. As a precaution, rinse vegetables thoroughly before peeling or cooking them. Another way you can acquire the illness is through raw or undercooked meat, especially pork.

Make sure to wash your hands after handling raw meat, and cook meat thoroughly.

Hot Tubs and Saunas

Q CAN I USE A HOT TUB OR SPA?

A The biggest concern about hot tubs is the temperature of the water and the core body temperature of the pregnant woman. It's important that your core body temperature stay below 102°F. When your body gets warmer than 102°F, your developing baby needs more oxygen and can get overheated. A second concern is the risk of getting an infection from bacteria in the water.

Because of concern about birth defects, especially neural tube defects, care providers recommend that women stay out of a hot tub during the first trimester. After that, many care providers still advise against it. Other providers say short stays are all right if you monitor your temperature with a thermometer. The best way to ensure that you don't overheat is to set the water temperature below 102°F. Checking with your care provider will make you more comfortable with your decision.

Q WHAT ABOUT SAUNAS?

A Most care providers advise against saunas. They're designed to run at a hot temperature, and you can overheat very quickly.

Environmental Toxins

Q WHAT PRECAUTIONS DO I NEED TO TAKE REGARDING LEAD?

A Lead is a metal that accumulates in the body and damages the nervous system, causing hearing, learning, and behavioral problems. Pregnant women, their developing babies, and young children are most at risk. The most common sources of lead are drinking water, lead paint, and ceramic ware.

Lead in drinking water most often comes from plumbing. Lead pipes are no longer used but may remain in buildings built before 1900. Most buildings built after 1900 have copper plumbing. The lead comes from the solder used to join the pipes. If the water is not corrosive, it takes about five years for the inside of the pipes to become coated with minerals found in the water. This coating prevents the lead from leaching into the water. Plastic (PVC) pipes do not contain lead. The best way to determine whether your water contains lead is to have it tested. Visit the Environmental Protection Agency website at www.epa.gov/safewater/lead/lead1.html or contact your local health department for information regarding water testing. If you get your water from a well, it's a good idea to have it tested periodically to make sure it hasn't become contaminated with environmental pollutants.

If you're worried about lead in your drinking water, you can minimize the threat of exposure by drinking or cooking only with water from the cold tap. Before using it, run the water until it's as cold as it can get. This flushes out the water that may have been in contact with lead.

Lead in paint was banned nationally in 1978. If you live in a building that was built after that, you don't have to worry about lead in paint chips or dust when you're remodeling or redecorating. If you live in a building that was built before then, you need to consider the risk of inhaling lead dust when you sand painted surfaces. To keep that lead out of your body and away from your developing baby, have someone else prepare the surfaces you want to repaint. Stay away until all floors and surfaces have been vacuumed and wiped with a damp cloth. Lead paint that has been painted over (and isn't flaking) is not a risk to you.

Earthenware or ceramic dishes may contain lead. If the item isn't certified lead free, consider using it for decoration only. At the very least, avoid putting acidic foods on the dishes. The acidity speeds up the leaching of the lead.

Q WHAT OTHER ENVIRONMENTAL CHEMICALS DO I NEED TO WORRY ABOUT?

A Most cleaning products used in the home are not a risk to you or your developing baby. However, make sure to read the label so you use the product appropriately. Wear gloves to protect your skin. If there's a strong smell, ventilate the area well. If the product smells too strong to you, have someone else use it.

One task you'll want to leave to others is applying pesticides, both indoors and out. Before beginning, cover anything that comes in contact with food. Indoors, ventilate the room after the pesticide has been applied. Stay away for at least several hours and have someone else wash off any food preparation surfaces.

If you work in a field that exposes you to chemicals, talk with your care provider about whether you need to take special precautions. The Occupational

Safety and Health Administration (OSHA) www.osha.gov and the National Institute for Occupational Safety and Health (NIOSH) www.cdc.gov/niosh/homepage.html are good places to research workplace safety.

Travel

Q How can I best protect my baby when I'm in a car?

A Wear your seat belt. It can save your life as well as your baby's. Position the lap portion low over your hips, below your belly. The shoulder portion should ride over your shoulder and chest. Buckle up every time you're in the car. A majority of accidents happen close to home.

In case you're in a crash, it's safest if there's a little distance between you and the part of the car that launches the front air bag. When you're driving, set the seat as far back as is comfortable for you. You want to be at least 10 inches from the steering wheel. If the steering column tilts, try having it tilt upward. When you're riding in the front seat as a passenger, slide the seat back as far as possible. (See page 141 for information about infant car seats.)

Q Can I travel while I'm pregnant?

A Most women can travel while they're pregnant. However, care providers usually recommend staying close to home in the last month or so. This is to minimize the chance of giving birth in an unplanned setting. Check with your provider before making a long trip to make sure there isn't a medical reason for rescheduling the trip. Here are some things you can do to increase your comfort while traveling:

- If you're flying, request an aisle seat. That will make getting up easier. A bulkhead seat usually gives you a little more legroom.
- Get up and walk around for a few minutes every hour or so. While you're up, use the bathroom. Avoid sitting for more than two hours at a time.
- Keep drinking water to prevent dehydration that can lead to premature labor and severe headaches.
- Eat small, healthy snacks.
- Use a small pillow to support your lower back.
- Do ankle circles (page 43) and stepping in place to help reduce swelling in your feet.
- If you're traveling by car, stop every hour or so. Walk around a bit and do some slow stretches to keep from getting stiff.

APPEARANCE

Q WHEN WILL I LOOK PREGNANT?

A How quickly your pregnancy shows depends on several factors including your height, prepregnancy weight, and clothing style. It may be five months before others notice any change, although you may feel your waistband getting tighter before then. If you're carrying twins or have been pregnant before, you'll likely show earlier. By six months a pregnancy is usually obvious.

Q WHEN I COMPARE HOW BIG I AM WITH HOW OTHER PREGNANT WOMEN LOOK, I DON'T SEEM TO BE THE RIGHT SIZE.

A Many women think they look too large or too small. Belly size depends a lot on body type and the way a woman is carrying her pregnancy. Tall women have a longer torso, so their abdomens may not stick out as far. Some babies seem to ride high while others look like they're heading for the woman's knees. Some women carry their pregnancy all out in front; others seem to have gotten wider all the way around. Your care provider will measure your uterus at prenatal visits and can reassure you about your growth.

Q CAN YOU TELL THE SEX OF THE BABY BY THE SHAPE OF THE MOTHER'S ABDOMEN?

A No, although there are a lot of myths linking the mother's appearance to her baby's sex. If knowing your baby's sex before birth is important to you, discuss this with your care provider. An ultrasound usually shows if the baby is a boy or girl.

Hair

Q MY HAIR HAS GOTTEN VERY THICK. HOW LONG WILL THIS LAST?

A The increased estrogen and faster metabolism of pregnancy make your hair grow faster than usual. Also, because your body retains hair longer, you end up with more hair, leading to the added thickness. You'll lose this excess hair during the first six months after the baby is born. Most women find their hair returns to the thickness and texture they had before pregnancy. Some, however, find their hair retains the change that started in pregnancy, remaining curlier, straighter, or a different color.

Q I THOUGHT A PREGNANT WOMAN'S HAIR IS SUPPOSED TO LOOK THICK AND RICH. MINE DOESN'T. WHAT HAPPENED?

A Unfortunately, not all hair changes are desirable. The hormones of pregnancy affect oil production in the skin and can create oilier hair than normal. If this is your situation, try using products made for oily hair. Sometimes curly hair goes limp or straight. Consider wearing your hair differently and using styling products that enhance your new look. These kinds of hair changes are not likely to persist after your baby is born.

Q CAN I CONTINUE TO COLOR MY HAIR THROUGHOUT MY PREGNANCY?

A There isn't enough research to make a definitive statement. Care providers have different opinions regarding the safety of hair dyes. The issue is whether the dye can harm the developing baby. Talk to your care provider so you can make a decision you'll be comfortable with. To minimize the negative effects of hair coloring:
- Wait until you're more than 12 weeks pregnant to have your hair colored. By that time all of your baby's systems will have been formed.
- Avoid having the coloring come in contact with your skin. This will prevent your system from absorbing the chemicals.
- Consider having your hair highlighted, frosted, or streaked. These techniques keep the color away from your scalp.
- Apply the color in a well-ventilated room to minimize inhalation of fumes.
- Consider using less permanent kinds of color to decrease the strength of the chemicals being used.
- Ask your stylist about using vegetable dyes.

Q CAN I STRAIGHTEN MY HAIR OR GET A PERMANENT WHEN I'M PREGNANT?

A There are two issues related to chemicals that either curl or relax hair. One is safety, and the other is result. The safety issue is the same as with hair coloring: the risk of chemicals harming your developing baby. Ask your care provider's advice. If you get a permanent or straighten your hair, use the suggestions above to reduce the risk of exposure to chemicals.

On the issue of results, some stylists advise against these procedures when you're pregnant because the outcome can be uneven or frizzy, or the process doesn't "take." Consider other ways to style your hair, or choose a cut that works with your straighter (or curlier) hair.

Skin Darkening

Q WHY ARE THERE DARK PATCHES OF SKIN AROUND MY EYES?

A During pregnancy, specific areas of skin get darker because of increased pigmentation. These can include the skin over your cheeks, nose, and forehead. It's called chloasma, or the mask of pregnancy. Exposure to the sun increases this darkening. After you give birth, these patches will slowly fade, although they may not totally disappear. To minimize this darkening:

- Wear sunscreen or sunblock whenever you go out in the sun.
- Wear a hat that shades your face.
- Wear makeup to minimize the different skin tones if the change is distressing.

Q WHY DO I HAVE A DARK LINE GROWING UP THE MIDDLE OF MY BELLY?

A Before you got pregnant, you probably didn't notice that you had a light line between your bellybutton and your pubic bone. It's called a linea alba. Starting in the third month, this line darkens on some women. It's then called a linea nigra. If this is your first baby, the darkening will grow toward your navel at about the same rate as the top of your uterus moving upward. In subsequent pregnancies, the entire line often appears at once. This darkening is part of the increased pigmentation that occurs during pregnancy. It will fade after your baby is born.

Spider Nevi

Q WHAT ARE THE REDDISH STAR-SHAPED MARKS THAT HAVE APPEARED ON MY UPPER BODY?

A These vascular spiders, called spider nevi, are small, dilated blood vessels in the skin. They commonly appear on the chest, arms, neck, and face and are easiest to see on light skin. The high level of estrogen stimulates the growth of these blood vessels, which are harmless and need no treatment. Usually they diminish after the baby is born, but may not disappear completely. A dermatologist can remove them after your baby is born if their visibility bothers you.

Q I HAVE SPIDER VEINS ON MY LEGS AND THIGHS. WILL THEY BECOME VARICOSE VEINS?

A No. Spider veins are not baby varicose veins. They're small blood vessels in the skin.

ACHES AND CONCERNS

Feeling Lightheaded

Q WHY DO I SOMETIMES FEEL LIGHTHEADED NOW THAT I'M PREGNANT?

A There are a few reasons why you may feel lightheaded or dizzy at times. One is that the hormones of pregnancy relax blood vessels. This has the effect of lowering blood pressure. It also makes it harder to keep blood in your head when you change positions quickly. Avoid moving suddenly from a lying down or sitting position to standing. Change your position slowly, especially if you've been lying down for a while.

Another cause may be dehydration. Your body needs at least eight cups of fluid a day. If it's hot or if you live in a dry climate, you may need even more. Keep a tumbler or travel mug of ice water nearby so you can sip it throughout the day.

A third cause may be low blood sugar. If you're having trouble with morning sickness, you may not be eating enough or frequently enough to keep your blood sugar at a normal level. Keep stashes of high-quality snacks such as fruit, whole-grain crackers, nuts, or protein bars at work, in your purse, and in your car. That way you can nibble on something whenever you need to. Contact your care provider if you have persistent dizziness or a bad headache along with feeling lightheaded.

Feeling Warm

Q NOW THAT I'M PREGNANT, I ALWAYS FEEL WARM.
WHAT'S CAUSING THAT?

A During pregnancy your metabolism speeds up. In addition, the increased amount of circulating blood warms your skin. As a result, you feel warm, even hot. This can be a benefit if it's cool outside. However, it makes heat harder to bear. Take precautions to prevent becoming over-heated. Avoid staying out in the hot sun. Exercise in an air-conditioned room or when the day is coolest.

Q I'M PERSPIRING A LOT MORE THAN I EVER DID.
WHAT CAN I DO ABOUT THAT?

A Perspiring is the normal, healthy reaction to increased body tempera-ture. The evaporating perspiration regulates your temperature. Dressing in layers can help you stay more comfortable. So can wearing clothes made from natural fibers (like cotton) that breathe rather than trap moisture against your skin. Keeping your room cool and taking lukewarm baths or showers can also help. Make sure to drink plenty of fluids so you don't get dehydrated.

The increased perspiration can cause skin problems like heat rash. Dusting with cornstarch or baby powder after you bathe can help keep your skin dry. Sometimes the skin in body creases can get red and glazed or become infected. If this happens, ask your care provider about the best way to treat the problem.

Stuffy Nose and Nosebleeds

Q WHY IS MY NOSE STUFFY ALL THE TIME?

A Pregnancy causes a major increase in your blood supply. This ensures that your circulatory system can meet your needs and those of your growing baby. Unfortunately, this can also cause the mucous membranes in your nose to swell. You may find some relief by sleeping with a humidifier in your bedroom and lingering in a steamy bathroom. Ask your care provider about using saline nose drops or a decongestant.

Q I'VE HAD SEVERAL NOSEBLEEDS. IS THAT NORMAL?

A In addition to a stuffy nose, some women get nosebleeds. These, too, are caused by swollen mucous membranes. A humidifier may help limit the number of nosebleeds. Putting a little petroleum jelly on the irritated area can also be helpful.

Excessive Salivation

Q WHY DO I HAVE A LOT MORE SALIVA THAN USUAL?

A Many women notice an excess of saliva in the first months of pregnancy. This may be related to morning sickness. Nausea causes increased swallowing that triggers saliva production. Eating dry starchy foods does, too. This problem usually disappears on its own by the end of the third month. Until it does, try using the mouth-drying properties of mint:
- Brush your teeth with a mint-flavored toothpaste.
- Swish with a minty mouthwash several times a day.
- Suck on breath mints or try chewing sugarless gum.

Skin Oiliness/Dryness

Q MY SKIN IS A LOT DIFFERENT NOW THAT I'M PREGNANT. WILL THESE CHANGES LAST?

A Probably not. The changes are related to the hormones of pregnancy and the increased amount of blood in your circulatory system. The extra blood makes the skin more supple and able to retain moisture better. The increased estrogen darkens freckles, slows oil production, and dries the skin. Some women find their skin is oilier; others find theirs drier than normal. The end result varies according to what kind of skin you had to begin with. This temporary change is likely to require changing skin products at least until after your baby is born.

Many women find they have less acne. It's very important that pregnant women stop taking oral acne medication like Retin-A or Accutane because these can harm a developing baby.

Q MY FACE IS A LOT OILIER THAN IT WAS.
WHAT CAN I DO ABOUT THAT?

A You may find it helpful to use a facial cleansing product designed for oily skin and an astringent lotion in the morning and at night. Make sure any makeup you use is oil free and formulated so that it won't clog your pores.

Q WHAT'S THE BEST THING TO DO FOR DRY SKIN?

A The best thing to do is keep your skin well moisturized:
• Use a moisturizing cleanser or body wash rather than soap.
• Take warm showers rather than long hot baths.
• Apply a moisturizer designed for dry skin while your skin is a little damp.
• Use a room humidifier.
• Drink plenty of water.

Hands and Nails

Q MY FINGERNAILS ARE QUITE DIFFERENT.
WHAT'S CAUSING THIS CHANGE?

A Pregnancy hormones are behind the changes in nails, which are apt to grow faster but are also more likely to be softer or more brittle. Sometimes grooves appear in the nails. These changes won't remain after the baby is born. For now, keeping your nails short may be best. Consider wearing gloves when you do housework or gardening. Also, make sure you're getting enough protein and calcium.

Q THE PALMS OF MY HANDS ARE RED AND ITCHY.

A It's common to have red, itchy palms during pregnancy. The soles of the feet can also be affected. Lotion may soothe some of the itching. The redness won't go away until after your baby is born because pregnancy hormones cause this condition.

Q MY RINGS ARE GETTING TIGHT.
HOW CAN I KEEP MY FINGERS FROM GETTING TOO BIG?

A Toward the end of pregnancy, many women find they can no longer wear their rings. The extra fluid they have in their bodies makes their fingers too large for the rings to fit comfortably. It's better to take your rings off when they start to get tight. That way you won't risk having to have them cut off by a jeweler. Keeping your weight gain within the target range can help with finger size. Make sure to keep all your prenatal appointments so your care provider can monitor your fluid retention. Contact your provider if you have severe swelling or any of the warning signs described on page 73.

Heartburn and Indigestion

Q WHAT'S CAUSING MY HEARTBURN?

A The increased amount of progesterone and the pregnancy hormone relaxin slow the emptying of your stomach. This makes it easier for stomach contents, which are acidic, to go up into your esophagus (the tube that connects your throat to your stomach.) That causes the burning feeling in your chest or the back of your throat. In addition, as your uterus grows larger, it crowds your stomach and can make the heartburn worse. There are things you can do to help prevent or relieve heartburn:

- Eat smaller, more frequent meals. This will limit the amount of food in your stomach.
- Avoid foods that trigger heartburn. Coffee and caffeinated beverages, fatty or fried foods, tomato sauce, and spicy foods are often culprits. Keeping a food diary will help you identify foods that are a problem for you.
- Remain upright after you eat. Squat rather than bend over at the waist. If you need to lie down within two hours after eating, prop your head and shoulders with pillows.
- When you do rest, lie on your side.
- Try raising the head of your bed on small blocks. This may reduce heartburn that comes during the night.
- Avoid wearing clothing that's tight around your middle.
- Ask your care provider to recommend an antacid, and follow the directions about how to take it. Avoid preparations that contain sodium. They can make you retain water and affect your blood pressure as well as cause swelling.
- Talk to your care provider if you experience a sudden increase in heartburn.

Q CAN THIS SLOWED EMPTYING OF MY STOMACH ALSO CAUSE INDIGESTION?

A Yes. The suggestions above for heartburn also work for indigestion. Whenever possible, avoid foods that cause you the most distress. If you also have bloating, ask your care provider to suggest a medication to relieve gas.

Abdominal Aches

Q I HAVE AN ACHE IN MY ABDOMEN THAT COMES AND GOES. IS THIS THE SIGN OF A MAJOR PROBLEM?

A Pregnancy brings many body changes that result in a variety of sensations. Because these sensations aren't familiar, they can be worrisome even if they're normal. You can call your care provider if you're concerned with how you're feeling.

There are several normal pregnancy changes that can cause an ache that comes and goes. As your uterus grows, it pulls on the ligaments that keep it anchored in your abdomen. This is especially true of the two round ligaments that are on the sides of your uterus. Later in pregnancy, these can cause a sharper, catching pain, especially if you quickly stretch upward. You may also be feeling your bladder. It can ache when it gets full because there isn't a lot of room for it and your uterus. The ache can also be from your large intestine. Food is moving through your intestines more slowly now, making constipation more likely.

Pains that are only on one side, are sharp or jabbing, or are intense, prolonged, or accompanied by bleeding should be immediately reported to your care provider. These are more apt to be signs of a problem. (See also pregnancy warning signs on page 73.)

Stretch Marks

Q WHAT CAN I DO TO PREVENT STRETCH MARKS?

A Some women have skin that's elastic enough to accommodate the changes of pregnancy without creating stretch marks, but most women don't. There isn't much you can do to prevent them. Stretch marks are the result of separations in the tissue just under the skin. This happens when a part of your body grows rapidly. Gaining weight slowly and steadily may minimize the number. Depending on your skin tone, the marks first appear as dark or purplish streaks. Over time they fade but never completely disappear. Body lotions or creams may make your skin feel a little better, but they won't prevent the stretch marks.

Constipation

Q WHY IS IT SO EASY TO GET CONSTIPATED WHEN YOU'RE PREGNANT? HOW CAN I PREVENT IT?

A The hormones of pregnancy, especially progesterone, slow the passage of food through your digestive tract. This allows your body to use more of the nutrients from the food. It also means you're more likely to get constipated. To keep things moving:

- Drink at least eight cups (64 ounces) of fluid each day.
- Eat at least five servings of fruits and vegetables each day.
- Try drinking prune juice or adding prunes to fruit or vegetable salads.
- Avoid bananas, which increase constipation.
- Choose whole grains like whole-wheat bread, brown rice, and whole-grain cereals.
- Read the nutrition labels of grain products to help you choose products that are high in fiber.
- Walk, swim, or bike at least half an hour each day. (See page 61.)

If these methods don't prevent constipation, talk to your care provider about:

- Changing formulations of any iron or calcium supplements and antacids you're taking. These can cause constipation.
- Using a supplement that contains psyllium to create bulk. It can be purchased either as capsules or crystals that are dissolved in water or juice.
- Using a stool softener if the other methods have failed. Avoid laxatives unless they're prescribed by your care provider.

Hemorrhoids

Q HOW CAN I PREVENT HEMORRHOIDS?

A Hemorrhoids are varicose veins in the anus. They can itch, burn, and bleed, making bowel movements very uncomfortable. The increased progesterone and pressure from the growing uterus make hemorrhoids a common problem. Constipation also makes hemorrhoids more likely and can make existing ones worse. Some women get hemorrhoids during pregnancy. Others get them from straining while pushing during labor. (See page 95 for a description of spontaneous pushing. This technique may minimize the risk of getting a hemorrhoid during childbirth.) Here are some things you can do to prevent hemorrhoids:

- Avoid constipation. (See page 41 for a list of suggestions.)
- Avoid prolonged straining when having a bowel movement.
- Avoid sitting on the toilet for long periods of time.

Q I'M SUFFERING FROM HEMORRHOIDS. WHAT CAN YOU SUGGEST?

A To reduce swelling, itching, and burning:

- Take a sitz bath (sit in a shallow bath) several times a day. Have the water be very warm.
- Soak cotton balls in witch hazel and freeze them. Then apply them to the area of the hemorrhoid.
- Use over-the-counter creams and suppositories like Preparation H and Anusol that are designed to bring comfort.
- Keep the area clean by gently wiping from front to back.
- Do Kegel exercises to improve circulation. (See pages 64–65.)
- If you're still miserable, ask your care provider about other treatments that may be appropriate.

Varicose Veins

Q I THINK I'M GETTING VARICOSE VEINS IN MY LEGS. WHAT CAN I DO?

A If varicose veins run in your family, you may get them during pregnancy. They can appear as early as the end of the second trimester. They're caused by pregnancy changes including an increased blood supply, relaxation of blood vessels, and a growing uterus. As it becomes harder for circulating blood to get back to the heart, it collects in the veins of the legs, making them swell. That results in varicose veins. Here are some things you can do:

- Avoid standing in one place for a long period of time. If you must stand, walk around as much as possible. Walking helps return blood to your heart.

- Do leg and foot exercises to improve circulation. These include ankle circles (see below) and foot pumps. While sitting, extend one leg and gently yet firmly flex your foot so you point your heel. This will make your toes move toward your body. Then relax your foot. Repeat this action ten times, then switch feet.
- Take a daily walk or swim a few laps.
- Put your feet up whenever possible.
- Avoid crossing your legs or wearing knee-highs that can constrict blood vessels.
- Consider wearing maternity stockings for their support. Maternity support stockings are also available. These are made of a heavier, stretchier material than regular stockings. They're best put on before you get out of bed in the morning.

Swollen Feet

Q MOST OF MY SHOES NO LONGER FIT COMFORTABLY. BY THE END OF THE DAY, MY ANKLES AND FEET ARE SWOLLEN. WHAT CAN I DO?

A As your belly and baby grow during the third trimester, you're likely to find your feet getting larger, too. This is partly due to swelling. It's harder for your heart to pump the blood out of your feet, especially while you're standing still. Also, because your joints are looser and your body is heavier, your feet actually get about a half size larger. To make yourself and your feet more comfortable:

- Work your legs and feet.
  * Take a walk or do any exercise that involves your legs and feet. Swimming is an excellent exercise to reduce swelling.
  * Do ankle circles throughout the day. Do a set by making ten circles with your feet going to the left and ten going to the right.
- Use gravity to reduce the swelling.
  * Sit with your feet up whenever you can. Try to do this for 15 minutes before you go to bed. That will allow you to sleep a little longer before having to get up to go to the bathroom.
  * Lie on the floor or on a sofa, and rest your feet on a large pillow, low chair, arm of the sofa, or against the wall. Your feet only have to be above the level of your heart. To avoid lying flat on your back, roll a little toward your left side. Use a pillow or rolled blanket to maintain your position.

- Invest in a new pair of comfortable shoes with low heels. You'll be able to wear the shoes after your baby is born, since your feet will likely remain a larger size.
- Get a pedicure. The foot massage will feel wonderful, and you'll like not having to struggle to cut your toenails.

Sleep Comfort

Q WHAT CAN I DO TO GET SOME SLEEP? I ONLY SLEEP A FEW HOURS A NIGHT BECAUSE I JUST CAN'T GET COMFORTABLE.

A As you get closer to giving birth, it gets harder and harder to sleep well at night. Loss of mobility and achy joints make getting into a comfortable position difficult. Some sleep accessories and a nighttime routine may help. To get your body more relaxed and comfortable before getting into bed:

- Take a warm shower and do some slow stretches to ease tension in your neck, shoulders, and back. Do a hula dance and sway your hips from side to side, forward and back, and in a circle.
- Take a warm bath and let the water relax your tired muscles. Have someone help you out of the tub, since a long bath can make you feel lightheaded.
- Do 10–15 minutes of yoga, then slip into bed for 10 minutes of relaxation breathing. (See pages 59–60.)

To help your bed support your body better:
- Put a foam "egg crate" pad under the bottom sheet.
- Use a sleeping bag to add a layer of softness between you and the mattress.
- Sleep against a body pillow to support your back while you're side lying.
- Use as many pillows as you need to support your belly, arms, and hips. Put a pillow between your knees.

If you wake up and can't get comfortable:
- Take a stroll around your home after you go to the bathroom.
- Rest in a reclining chair.

FEARS AND FEELINGS

Emotional Swings

Q WHAT'S THE MATTER WITH ME? ONE MINUTE I FEEL GREAT AND THE NEXT MINUTE I CAN'T STOP FROM BURSTING INTO TEARS.

A The hormones that cause the physical changes in pregnancy also affect your emotions. The intensity of your emotional shifts may vary during the course of your pregnancy. Most women find the widest swings during the first trimester when the body and mind are trying to get used to being pregnant. The second trimester is often the calmest. Then, the emotional swings are likely to increase again during the third trimester. Having a baby may be the greatest change in a woman's life. It's not surprising, then, that you'd feel a range of emotions.

Q **I WANTED THIS PREGNANCY VERY MUCH. BUT NOW THAT I'M PREGNANT, I'M NOT SO SURE. DOES THIS MEAN I'M NOT GOING TO BE A GOOD MOTHER?**

A Not at all. It means that being a good mother is important to you. Many women have periods of mixed or even negative feelings after they find out they're pregnant. As you consider all that motherhood involves, you may not feel ready. However, women grow into motherhood. Most women feel more confident as the pregnancy progresses. Consider sharing your feelings with your partner or a trusted friend. This may help you put things in perspective.

Q **IT SEEMS EVERYWHERE I TURN THERE'S A STORY OR PICTURE OF A BABY WITH A PROBLEM. WHY DO I FEEL SO VULNERABLE?**

A It's normal to want to protect your baby. This heightens your awareness of messages about danger, especially danger to babies. However, knowing that your feelings are normal may not be comforting to you. Remember that very few babies are born with serious problems. If you're worried about a specific problem, share this with your care provider. There may be a way to reassure you. If you're the kind of person who feels better if you have a plan, make one. Planning for a problem will not cause it to happen.

Q **I'VE STRUGGLED WITH DEPRESSION IN THE PAST, AND I'M WORRIED THAT IT WILL RETURN.**

A A woman can suffer from depression during pregnancy, and a previous episode increases the risk. It also increases the risk of postpartum depression. (See pages 142–144.) Tell your care provider about your history and current concerns. Together you can monitor how you're feeling and take action if necessary. Depression responds to treatment. Consider seeing a therapist who has experience dealing with prenatal and postpartum depression. In addition, develop a support network if you don't already have one. It's important that you don't feel alone.

Q PEOPLE I DON'T EVEN KNOW COME UP AND GIVE ME ADVICE. SOMETIMES IT'S OKAY, BUT OTHER TIMES I FEEL OVERWHELMED BY WHAT THEY'RE TELLING ME. WHAT CAN I DO?

A People sometimes feel free to approach a pregnant woman and say or do things they wouldn't say or do to anyone else. This invasion of your privacy and personal space may be annoying—or worse. How you respond depends on your personality and how you feel at the moment. Some women try to cut the person off with an ironic, funny, or even sharp remark. Others respond by saying, "I don't need to hear that just now," and walk away. Don't feel obligated to hear the person out.

Dreaming and Forgetfulness

Q I KEEP FORGETTING THINGS. WHY CAN'T I CONCENTRATE?

A Forgetfulness during pregnancy is not a sign of decreased mental ability. It's a sign of all that's happening. You have a lot to think about when you're pregnant: your developing baby, being a parent, and your other responsibilities. As a result, you're not always focused on the task at hand. To help you with this temporary forgetfulness:

- Get as much rest as you can. Being overtired makes it harder to keep focused.
- Use relaxation techniques to reduce your stress. Stress can make you more forgetful.
- Write notes to yourself and post them where you can see them.
- Use a calendar, daily planner, or PDA (personal digital assistant) to keep track of commitments and deadlines. Check this reminder frequently.
- Before going into a meeting or starting a new task, stop and take a deep breath. Focus on what you're about to do.

Q I FIND MYSELF DAYDREAMING A LOT. DO OTHER PREGNANT WOMEN DO THAT?

A Yes. Daydreaming is part of the important work of pregnancy. Becoming a mother brings immense changes in your life and how you view yourself. Daydreaming helps you process that change. You'll probably spend a lot of time looking back at how you were parented and your family relationships. This is part of exploring what kind parent you want to be. In addition, you may dream about your baby. As your pregnancy advances, your baby will play an even greater role in stimulating your daydreaming about what he or she will be like.

Q MY DREAMS ARE OFTEN VIVID AND INTENSE. IS THIS NORMAL?

A Pregnant women can have very intense dreams that may involve vivid colors and dramatic action. Some can be quite erotic. Sometimes the dreams can be disturbing because they're about not being a good parent or about a baby with a problem. These dreams are not omens. They're part of getting ready for whatever lies ahead. Telling your partner or a trusted friend about an especially vivid dream may help you feel less overwhelmed by the images.

Maternal Ties

Q I SEEM TO BE SPENDING A LOT OF TIME THINKING ABOUT MY MOTHER.

A During pregnancy women explore what it means to be a mother. This involves a lot of thinking about their own mothers, which can generate both positive and negative feelings. Most women think of ways they want to be like their mothers and things they want to do differently.

Becoming a mother adds a new dimension to a woman's relationship with her mother. If your mother is available, pregnancy provides an opportunity to deepen that relationship. If your mother has died or is not available, you might feel great sadness or anger about her not being with you. Finding a way to express your feelings can be helpful. Tell her by writing her a letter or imagining she's sitting in a chair opposite you.

YOUR PARTNER'S HEALTH HABITS

Q HOW IMPORTANT ARE MY PARTNER'S HEALTH HABITS?

A A man's health can affect sperm production. If you're already pregnant, this will no longer be an issue. However, your family's health is. If you're making a lifestyle change such as quitting smoking or avoiding alcohol, it will be easier to stick with this change if your partner's lifestyle supports it. In addition, your partner's food preferences affect the family's diet and will influence your child's food choices.

If your partner does not want to make a change with you, find a family member or friend who can support the choice you're making. When you find it difficult to sustain your change, you will have someone who can give you encouragement.

MOVING TOWARD PARENTHOOD

Q ALTHOUGH MY PARTNER WAS THRILLED WHEN WE LEARNED I WAS PREGNANT, HE HASN'T MENTIONED THE PREGNANCY FOR A WEEK. WHAT'S THE MATTER?

A The fact that your partner hasn't mentioned the pregnancy is not a sign of rejection. Because you're the one who is pregnant, you can't forget that you are. Your partner, on the other hand, can. Although expectant parents do similar types of things to prepare for parenthood, they have different timelines. Many expectant partners talk of being glad pregnancy lasts nine months because they need that much time to get ready.

Communication is the key to maintaining your relationship as you approach parenthood. Making time for each other can be especially challenging in the first few months after your baby is born. Starting now, set aside some quiet time to share your thoughts and concerns at least once a week. Establishing this habit during pregnancy will also help you after the baby is born.

Q I DON'T KNOW WHAT'S THE MATTER WITH MY PARTNER. HE'S GAINED MORE WEIGHT THAN I HAVE AND IS TIRED ALL THE TIME.

A It sounds like your partner may have Couvade Syndrome ("sympathetic pregnancy"). Many partners start having some of the same physical changes that are seen in pregnant women. In addition to weight gain and fatigue, these may include food cravings, nausea, vomiting, toothache, headache, dizziness, and mood swings. These tend to decrease after the third month but may reappear in the eighth month. They disappear after the baby is born.

There are several possible reasons for Couvade, including identification with the pregnancy, an increase in female hormones, anxiety, and jealousy. It's not something your partner is doing on purpose. Ask your partner to get a checkup to make sure he or she is in good health. That way neither of you will worry needlessly.

Q MY PARTNER DECIDED THAT WE NEED MORE INCOME TO RAISE OUR BABY, SO HE'S LOOKING FOR A SECOND JOB. I FEEL NEGLECTED. HOW CAN I GET HIM TO PAY MORE ATTENTION TO ME?

A In our society fathers have traditionally had the role of providing for their families. Your partner is taking on the role of being a good parent by being a good provider. This, however, leaves little time for the two of you. Make time for both of you to share your concerns. Perhaps you can go over your budget together and decide how much income is necessary. Knowing that your partner isn't trying to avoid you may make you feel less neglected.

Q NOW THAT MY PARTNER CAN FEEL THE BABY KICK, HE'S STARTED SPENDING MORE TIME BY HIMSELF. I'M AFRAID HE MAY NOT LIKE THE BABY.

A It's more likely that because he can feel the baby, being a father seems more real to him. It's common for fathers to turn inward at this time. Mothers usually turn inward earlier, in the third month of pregnancy.

Expectant fathers and mothers worry about their ability to be good parents. They think about how they were parented and how they want to parent. Your partner's preoccupation and quietness may not be the sign of a problem. If you want to begin a conversation about parenting, consider these topics:

- Things you liked about how your parents raised you;
- Things you want to do differently;
- Things you've seen other parents do that you'd like to try;
- Things your partner does that will make him or her a good parent.

Q ARE THERE OTHER PARENTING ISSUES WE SHOULD DISCUSS BEFORE THE BABY IS BORN?

A You and your partner may have different ideas about parenting, many of which come from how you were raised. Discussing these issues before the birth will show you where you agree and will identify items you need to discuss further. Although you'll need to adapt your parenting philosophy to fit your baby's needs, it's important that you both feel comfortable with basic parenting behaviors. Here are some questions to consider:

- How will we feed the baby?
- Where will the baby sleep?
- How quickly should we respond to our crying baby?
- What's the most important thing to accomplish in the first month?
- How much time will we take off from work or school?
- How will we share parenting responsibilities?
- How will we involve grandparents and other family members?

Q **MY PARTNER JUST WENT OUT AND BOUGHT A SET OF TOOLS TO MAKE SOMETHING FOR THE BABY. I'VE NEVER SEEN THIS SIDE OF HIM. WHAT'S GOING ON?**

A Expectant partners can have a burst of creativity as the baby's birth approaches. Some partners create songs or poems. Others make things with their hands. They also get a nesting instinct similar to expectant mothers. They want to prepare a space for the baby. See it as another positive sign of your partner's journey toward parenthood.

Q **I'M DUE IN A MONTH AND I'M TIRED AND ANXIOUS ABOUT BEING READY FOR THE BABY. HOWEVER, MY PARTNER WANTS US TO DO THINGS ALMOST EVERY NIGHT. HOW CAN I BE SOCIAL WITHOUT BECOMING AN EXHAUSTED WRECK?**

A Your partner probably realizes that it'll be a lot harder to maintain a social life after the baby is born. As a result, there's pressure to squeeze in dinners with friends as well as go to movies, concerts, or sporting events. It's easy for a pressured social life to collide with your need to rest and prepare for your baby. To better balance your energy and your partner's social demands:

- Sit down together and identify the most important things you want to do before the baby is born.
- Mark all your engagements on a calendar. Make sure to include work commitments, prenatal visits, and other demands on your time.
- Arrange for resting days before and after the most taxing commitments.
- Make sure you've set aside time for just the two of you.

- Simplify your entertaining by hosting a potluck or by ordering takeout instead of cooking.
- Combine two activities and go with friends to see a movie or an event.

YOUR SEXUAL RELATIONSHIP

Q NOW THAT I'M PREGNANT, I JUST DON'T FEEL THAT INTERESTED IN SEX. IS THIS NORMAL?

A Many women experience a drop in their sex drive during the first trimester. Nausea, sore breasts, and exhaustion can put a damper on sex. You'll probably feel considerably better in the second trimester, which may perk up your interest. If you've been trying hard to get pregnant, you may want a break from the focus on intercourse. Or, you may feel that now that you're pregnant, sex isn't as important as it was when you were trying to get pregnant.

Instead of focusing on sex, concentrate on communicating with your partner. One thing you can try is making a list of things your partner does that demonstrate love for you. Have your partner do the same. Then, set aside some time to share your lists. You may be surprised by what your partner values. Then, each of you ask for something from your list. That way you can both enjoy sharing your love.

Another thing to try is turning out the lights and eating by candlelight. While enjoying a leisurely dinner together, share how you're feeling. Listen to your partner's feelings and fears. This type of sharing increases intimacy, which over time may enhance your sex life.

Q I'M JUST TOO UNCOMFORTABLE FOR INTERCOURSE. WHAT ELSE COULD WE TRY?

A You and your partner can do other things that bring each other physical pleasure. Make sure to tell one another what feels good and what doesn't.
- Kiss, cuddle, and caress each other.
- Take turns smoothing massage oil or lotion on each other.
- Give each other a massage.
- Finger-paint on each other's body using bath gel, and then shower it off together.
- Perform oral sex or masturbate each other.

Q MY PARTNER ISN'T THAT INTERESTED IN SEX ANYMORE. WHAT COULD BE THE MATTER?

A It's not unusual for a partner's interest in sex to change during pregnancy. If you had been trying to get pregnant for a while, sex now may remind your partner of the tension during that time. Your partner may be afraid of hurting the baby or disrupting the pregnancy. Or, your partner may be afraid of hurting you. Some partners have trouble adapting to the changing shape of a pregnant woman's body. Others begin to see their pregnant partner as a mother and find it difficult to be sexual. Some partners get depressed during pregnancy, which can affect sexual functioning.

Set aside some quiet time to talk about how each of you feels. Consider using some of the suggestions from the preceding questions to stay close. In addition to talking to each other, suggest that your partner talk with other expectant and new fathers. (See page 140 for information about finding a Dad and Baby class.) If your partner is depressed, encourage him or her to seek counseling.

Q MY PARTNER WANTS TO HAVE SEX BUT IS AFRAID HE'LL HURT THE BABY. WHAT SHOULD I TELL HIM?

A Unless your care provider has told you not to have intercourse and to avoid orgasm, it's safe to have sex. Your baby is well protected in the womb surrounded by amniotic fluid. Although your baby may be able to feel the rhythmic contractions of your orgasm, your baby won't know you're having sex. Perhaps spending some time pleasuring one another without intercourse will make sex easier for your partner.

If you're in your third trimester, you may not be comfortable having the baby between you. Consider positions such as side-lying with your partner behind you, you on top, or you on your hands and knees.

Q I'VE NEVER ENJOYED SEX AS MUCH AS I AM NOW. WHAT'S CHANGED?

A You may feel a sense of freedom now that you don't have to worry about getting pregnant. The larger breasts and rounded shape of pregnancy may make you feel sexier. In addition, your partner's response to your new shape may be a turn-on. Another pregnancy change is increased blood flow to the vagina. This engorgement can heighten sexual response and make orgasm easier.

DOMESTIC VIOLENCE

Q MY PARTNER HAS BEEN TREATING ME ROUGHLY NOW THAT I'M PREGNANT. I DON'T KNOW WHAT TO DO.

A Expecting a baby can strain a relationship. Women who are in abusive relationships are at risk for domestic violence when they're pregnant. When domestic violence occurs, infants and children also become victims. No one deserves to be hurt emotionally or physically. You deserve some help to decide what's best for you and your baby.

Even if you're not ready to disclose what's happening in your life, you can still take action. Tell your care provider that you're living under a lot of strain. Pregnant victims of abuse are at risk for having a baby born too early or too small. Your care provider may monitor your health and your baby's health more closely, which may make it easier to talk more openly.

Look for signs that the clinic or practice is especially sensitive to domestic violence. Look for information in the waiting room, examining room, or bathroom that talks about domestic or intimate partner abuse. Sometimes staff members wear buttons that say, "We talk about family violence here." This may make it easier for you to talk about what's happening. The staff will be able to refer you to an agency that can help you.

You can also get information anonymously by visiting the National Domestic Violence Hotline website at www.ndvh.org or by calling 800-799-SAFE (7233). Or, you can call a local agency listed in the yellow pages under "Social and Human Services, Domestic Violence."

THE PLACENTA, MEMBRANES, AND AMNIOTIC FLUID

Q WHERE DOES THE PLACENTA COME FROM?

A By the time the fertilized egg implants in the wall of the uterus, it's a hollow ball of cells. Some of these cells become the placenta.

Q WHAT EXACTLY DOES THE PLACENTA DO?

A The placenta has two main roles. It helps maintain the pregnancy by secreting hormones like estrogen and progesterone. In addition, it transfers oxygen and nutrients to the baby, and transfers the baby's waste products (such as carbon dioxide) to the mother. The placenta does not usually act as a barrier against harmful substances. Chemicals like nicotine and alcohol cross the placenta, as do viruses.

Q WHERE DOES THE AMNIOTIC FLUID COME FROM?

A Fetal membranes extending from the placenta create the bag of water. Cells of the inner membrane create the fluid. New fluid is always being created. In addition, the baby drinks the fluid and the baby's kidneys produce urine, which the baby pees back into the fluid. That contributes to the production and circulation of the fluid. By around 38 weeks there are about 2 pints of amniotic fluid.

Q WHAT DOES THE AMNIOTIC FLUID DO?

A For one thing, amniotic fluid is a baby's exercise pool. Because the baby floats in it, all parts of the baby's body can develop symmetrically. Moving in the fluid helps build the baby's muscles. In addition, amniotic fluid helps the baby's urinary tract development. The baby drinks the fluid and urinates into it. The fluid also stimulates the baby's sense of taste, since it picks up flavors from the foods the mother eats.

In addition, the fluid helps the baby maintain a constant body temperature and helps protect the baby by cushioning against bumps and minor falls. However, if you suffer a direct blow to the belly or are in a car accident, notify your care provider immediately. During labor the amniotic fluid helps cushion the baby's head during contractions and may help dilate the cervix.

MOVEMENT AND STATES

Q WHEN WILL I BE ABLE TO FEEL MY BABY MOVE?

A Quickening (the awareness of the baby's movement) usually happens between the 16th and 20th week. If this is your first baby, it may take a while to identify these butterfly-light sensations. As your baby grows, these movements are easier to feel. Quickening may make you feel more like you *are* having a baby. It will take a little longer until your partner is able to share in the excitement and feel the baby's movements through your belly.

Q SOMETIMES MY BABY IS VERY ACTIVE, AND SOMETIMES SHE DOESN'T MOVE AT ALL. WHAT'S GOING ON?

A Babies in the womb go through periods of sleep and activity. They have their own sleep/wake cycle. Your baby's movements and activity level indicate what state she's in. When your baby is asleep, she's in one of two sleep states. In quiet sleep there's very little movement. Your baby usually doesn't respond to sounds or activity outside the womb. In active sleep she may move and stretch but isn't likely to be responsive.

When your baby is awake, she's either in the quiet alert or active alert state. During the quiet alert state you'll be able to feel her move, even explore. This is when she's attentive and may even play with you. (See pages 56–57.) In the active alert state there's a lot of activity. Your own activity or rest may not affect her vigorous movements.

Q HOW DOES MY BABY'S STATE RELATE TO FETAL MOVEMENT COUNTS?

A Many times expectant women are asked to spend time each day paying attention to their baby's movements. This is because a baby's movements show that the baby is getting a good supply of oxygen and nutrients from the placenta. The amount of activity a woman can feel varies during the pregnancy. You can ask your care provider about how much movement to expect from your baby each day.

You may be asked to pay attention to your baby's movements two times every twenty-four hours, and record whether you can feel at least four movements in an hour. It takes a lot longer to get four movements when the baby is asleep. Being aware of your baby's sleep/wake cycles can help you choose a time when your baby is awake. In addition, knowing more about your baby's activity may make movement counting an anticipated opportunity to interact with your baby.

Q DO MY BABY'S MOVEMENTS GIVE CLUES ABOUT WHAT HE'LL BE LIKE?

A A baby's movements can provide some clues. How easily he startles, the amount of activity, and the types of movements are all clues to your baby's temperament. Daydreaming and imagining what your baby will be like are normal and positive experiences during pregnancy.

Q SOMETIMES I THINK MY BABY GETS THE HICCUPS. DOES THAT HAPPEN?

A Yes, babies do get hiccups in the womb. As you've experienced, there's nothing you need to do. The hiccups stop by themselves.

Q MY PARTNER WANTS TO INTERACT WITH OUR BABY. IS THERE A GAME THEY CAN PLAY?

A Your developing baby is aware of your partner even though they can't see each other yet. You can take advantage of your baby's responsiveness by playing the following game after the 35th week of pregnancy. Choose a time when your baby is awake but not extremely active. Sit comfortably in a chair with your partner nearby so he or she can touch your belly.

Have your partner start by talking to your baby so your baby knows your partner is there. Then, have your partner very gently press on your belly near the baby's hand or foot. You can help find a good spot. Wait for 15 seconds to see if the baby responds. Many times a baby will respond by pushing out a hand or kicking a foot. Your partner may have to repeat the gentle pressing a couple of times before getting a response.

Once the baby reacts, they can play a short game of tag by responding to what the other has done. Your baby won't play for a long time, or may not play at all this time. However, when your baby does play, a round of prenatal tag can be a lot of fun.

Your partner can also talk or sing to your baby. You'll need to alert your partner to when your baby is awake. After you're in a comfortable position, have your partner get close. He needs to talk or sing loudly enough to be heard across the room. If your partner puts his hand on your belly, he may be able to feel the baby move in response to his voice.

SIGHT AND HEARING

Q CAN BABIES HEAR BEFORE THEY'RE BORN?

A Yes, they can hear from about 24 weeks. Babies constantly hear their mother's heartbeat. That's why the sound of a heartbeat can quiet a newborn. They also hear their mother's voice whenever she speaks. Babies get used to the environmental sounds they hear in the womb. That's why after birth babies may sleep through a dog barking, traffic noises, or other familiar sounds.

Q WILL MY BABY KNOW MY VOICE AT BIRTH?

A Yes. From birth babies will turn toward the sound of their mother's voice. Newborns can also recognize the voices of other family members and often turn toward the person when he or she speaks.

Q DOES MY BABY KNOW WHAT I'M SAYING?

A Developing babies and newborns do not understand words. However, they do respond to the rhythm and tone of a person's voice. They prefer the sound of pleasant speech.

Q SHOULD I READ OR TALK TO MY BABY BEFORE BIRTH?

A In the last trimester some parents spend time talking to their babies. Others feel no need to do so. Do whatever feels best to you. Your daily routine will provide the sounds and conversation your baby needs for development.

Newborns remember sound patterns they heard repeatedly in the womb. Some parents create a special time with their developing baby by reading a poem or story or singing a song. If you want, you can begin this activity any time after the sixth month. Although many parents choose a soothing song, choose whatever you like. Sit quietly for a few minutes each evening and recite a poem or sing a song. This will be a time when you feel closer to your baby.

After the birth, your baby will respond by quieting and listening when she hears the familiar poem or song. You may be able to use it to soothe your baby. It may also work as part of your baby's sleep-time routine.

Q WHEN CAN A DEVELOPING BABY SEE?

A Babies see from the seventh month of pregnancy. Your baby can see diffused light through your abdomen. On a warm bright day, pull up your shirt and let the sun shine directly on your belly. If your baby is in a quiet alert state, you may be able to feel his movements in response to the sunlight. You can also shine a small flashlight on your belly. Move the beam from side to side and feel your baby respond.

If you want to track your baby's sensory development, you can check out week-by-week development charts such as the one at www.pregnancy.about.com/cs/pregnancycalendar/l/blwbw.htm. Some of the most famous pictures of developing babies can be seen in *A Child Is Born* by Lennart Nilsson.

RELEASING STRESS POINTS

Q **BY THE END OF THE DAY, I OFTEN HAVE A PAIN AT THE BASE OF MY NECK THAT MY DOCTOR SAYS IS STRESS RELATED. WHAT CAN I DO TO GET SOME RELIEF?**

A Most people have a stress collection point, or a part of the body that gets tense first and stays tense the longest. Many people carry stress in their shoulders and necks. Others carry it in their lower backs. Pregnancy increases the physical strain on your muscles and joints. This, added to the stress of everyday life, can make you feel achy as well as tense.

To work on your stress collection point, sit in a chair that allows you to sit upright with your feet firmly on the floor. Starting at your feet, pay attention to how each part of your body feels. Stop any time something feels uncomfortable. Move that part a bit to see if you can get it into a more comfortable position. Then take in a full breath. In your mind direct your exhalation to that part of your body. Some people find it easier to use their inhalation. Do what feels best. Take your time and repeat the breath if you don't feel a positive change.

Slowly move up through your body, breathing into any part that feels tense. When you reach your head, take five deep breaths and let each one out slowly. Enjoy the reduced level of stress in your body.

You can also do this while lying on your side or relaxing in a warm bath. In the shower, you can direct the flow of water to coincide with your focused breathing.

RELAXATION BREATHING

Q **IS THERE A QUICKER WAY TO GET RELAXED THAN LYING DOWN AND LISTENING TO SOFT MUSIC?**

A Slow breathing by itself is a route to relaxation. All you need to do is find the depth of breathing that feels best. To find your level, sit comfortably or lie down and put your hands just below your waist. Slowly breathe in, taking your breath down to your hands. Continue breathing like this for about a minute. Consider how that feels.

Next, move your hands to below your belly. Bring your breath all the way down to your hands. Breathe at this level for about a minute. Do you like that level of breathing better?

If neither level feels easy and relaxing, try moving your hands up a bit to the level of your bellybutton. Once you've found the level you like best, you can go right to it. Let your breathing stay even and easy. After a few minutes, you'll begin to feel relaxed.

IMAGERY

Q HOW CAN I USE IMAGERY TO GET RELAXED?

A When you sit or lie quietly and concentrate on a relaxing scene, your body will relax. There are several ways to do this. One way is for someone to describe a scene to you. As you listen to the description, imagine yourself being there. Even though you're not paying attention to your muscles, you'll begin to relax.

Another way is to imagine a restful scene without someone describing it. Think of a location that you find appealing, such as a beach or the bank of a stream. Use all of your senses to imagine the details. What can you see, hear, smell, touch, and taste? An audiotape or CD of nature sounds may aid your imagination.

A third way is to recall a favorite, comforting place and go there in your mind. Your body will remember how that place makes you feel, and you'll begin to relax.

PREGNANCY ADAPTATIONS

Q WHY SHOULD I EXERCISE DURING PREGNANCY?

A Exercise can give you more energy and help you sleep better. It can improve your sense of well-being by decreasing tension and releasing hormones that decrease pain and give you a lift. Exercise can also increase your strength and stamina.

Q EXERCISE IS AN IMPORTANT PART OF MY LIFE. WHAT HAPPENS NOW THAT I'M PREGNANT?

A Most pregnant women can continue their noncompetitive sports and exercise routines with only a few modifications. However, pregnancy is a time to avoid activities that pose a significant risk of falling, like down-hill skiing and horseback riding, and that could affect oxygen intake, like scuba diving. Discuss your exercise plans with your care provider. That way you can make sure that there are no reasons to limit your activity.

As your pregnancy advances, you'll need to modify your routine. That can mean going at a slower pace or going a shorter distance. As your center of gravity changes, you may want to alter your activity, such as shifting to a stationary bike.

Q WHAT SHOULD I PAY ATTENTION TO WHEN I EXERCISE?

A Your body works harder at rest when you're pregnant than when you're not pregnant. As a result, you don't want to stress your body to an extreme. You can tell how well your body is doing by monitoring your breathing. If you can talk while you're exercising, your pace is fine. You also need to avoid getting dehydrated and overheated. In addition, the hormones of pregnancy affect your joints. To prevent injury, it's important to avoid jarring and pounding movements. (See page 62 for an exercise checklist.)

Q I'VE NEVER DONE MUCH EXERCISING. WHAT COULD I DO NOW THAT I'M PREGNANT?

A One of the best things you can do is start walking each day. Check with your care provider to make sure you have no restrictions. Then put on a pair of comfortable shoes and walk. Thirty minutes a day is a good goal to aim for. Here are some walking tips:

- Bring a water bottle and take frequent sips.
- Get a friend to walk with you. If you can carry on a conversation, you aren't walking too fast.
- If the weather is hot, walk early in the morning or in the evening.
- If you don't have a safe place to walk or the weather is bad, consider walking in a mall. Malls often open early for walkers.

If you have access to a pool, consider swimming. Because the water supports your weight, you don't have to worry about overstressing joints or straining muscles. In addition to working lots of muscles, swimming can prevent or reduce swelling in your legs.

Exercise Checklist

- If your sport recommends safety equipment, like a helmet, use it.
- Wear comfortable clothing and a bra that gives you good support.
- Start with a warm-up period to slowly increase your heart rate and breathing.
- Make sure you're not too winded to talk while exercising.
- Avoid getting overheated.
- Drink water before, during, and after your exercise, to prevent dehydration.
- Avoid jumping and jerky movements that can hurt your joints and ligaments.
- Listen to your body and modify your activity or stop entirely if you start feeling fatigue or discomfort.
- If your lower back is sore after exercising, contract your abdominal muscles during the next session so that you tuck in your buttocks. If this is your second or third baby, consider wearing a pregnancy support belt.
- End with a cool-down period to let your heart rate and breathing return to normal.
- Contact your medical provider if you have pain, persistent rapid heart rate or breathlessness, lightheadedness or dizziness, headache, difficulty walking, nausea and vomiting, or bleeding.
- Eat a healthy snack to replace the calories you burned while exercising.
- Avoid infrequent exercise that can lead to injury. Aim for an exercise schedule of 20–30 minutes at least three or four times a week.

SHOULDER CIRCLES AND REACHES

Q **WHAT EXERCISES WILL MAKE MY SHOULDERS AND UPPER BACK FEEL BETTER?**

A Increased breast size and hunching your shoulders can result in a nagging soreness. Be aware of your posture and concentrate on standing tall and sitting up straight. In addition, try these exercises, doing three sets a day:
- Gently rotate your shoulders in a large circle, moving first up and back for five circles. Then reverse the direction and do five more circles. You can do these in the shower or whenever you feel tense.
- Gently stretch your upper back by doing alternating reaches. Sit comfortably on the floor or in a chair. Adjust your position so you're sitting as tall as you can. Raise both arms so they're at the height of your shoulders. Slowly raise your right hand as high as it will go. Feel the stretch in your back. Lower your right hand and reach high with your left. Alternate hands for a total of ten reaches.

PELVIC TILT AND ROCK

Q **I'M BEGINNING TO GET AN ACHE IN MY LOWER BACK. IS THERE AN EXERCISE I CAN DO TO REDUCE THIS ACHE?**

A Weakened abdominal muscles contribute to back discomfort. You can improve muscle tone by doing the pelvic tilt. In addition, the motion of using the tilt to rock your pelvis often brings comfort. This exercise can be done in a number of positions.

If you're in your first trimester, it may be easier to learn this exercise lying on a firm surface. Lie on your back with your knees bent and the soles of your feet flat on the floor. Tighten your abdominal muscles and tilt your pelvis in order to press the small of your back against the floor. Hold that position for the count of five and then relax. Repeat ten times. Once you feel confident that you know how to do the pelvic tilt, you can do it in other positions. Choose the one that feels best to you.

If you're more than four months pregnant, it's better not to lie on your back. Instead, start with a standing position. Stand straight and bend your knees just a bit so your pelvis is free to move. Contract your stomach muscles and tuck in your buttocks. This will rotate your pelvis and flatten your back. Hold that position for the count of five and then relax. Repeat ten times.

You can also do this exercise on hands and knees. In this position, avoid letting the small of your back sag. That will add to your backache. Instead, just return to a neutral position when you're relaxing out of the tilt. This position can also be helpful when you're in labor. Some women prefer to do pelvic tilts while sitting on a firm chair.

For pelvic rocking, smoothly do a series of pelvic tilts. Make the time in the tilt position and relaxed position about the same. You can do this anytime you want. If you want to add breathing, inhale in the relaxed position and exhale during the tilt.

POSTURE

Q NOW THAT MY BELLY IS LARGE, I FEEL A BIT OFF BALANCE AND MY BACK OFTEN ACHES. HOW CAN I IMPROVE MY POSTURE?

A As your abdomen gets large and sticks out, your center of gravity begins to shift. That usually results in leaning back from the waist in an attempt to compensate for this shift. It's very common to see a pregnant woman leaning back and putting a hand on the back of her hip. This posture can add to the stress on the back. You may find it more comfortable to focus on standing tall. Use a bit of a pelvic tilt to counter the weight of your uterus pulling your pelvis forward. (See page 63.)

You can check your posture by standing with your back against a wall. If there's a space of more than a hand's width at the small of your back, do a pelvic tilt to reduce that space. Stand that way until you can feel the difference in your posture. Although you may not be able to maintain a pelvic tilt while you're walking, try to return to your standing tall posture whenever you're standing or sitting. If you're going to stand in one place for a period of time, put one foot up on a small box or large phone book. That will help you keep your pelvic tilt. Move around a bit and alternate feet every 15 minutes or so.

SUPER KEGEL

Q SOMETIMES WHEN I COUGH OR LAUGH, I LEAK A LITTLE URINE. WHAT CAN I DO TO PREVENT THIS?

A Between your pubic bone and spine you have muscles that form a sling that supports your uterus and other pelvic organs. Within this group of muscles are those that control the flow of urine. These muscles can lose tone because of the increased size and weight of your uterus. Kegel exercises work these muscles and can maintain or improve their tone.

The best way to identify these muscles is to start the flow of urine and then stop it. The muscles you've tightened to stop the flow are the ones you need to exercise. Once you've identified these muscles, you should not start and stop the flow of urine as an exercise.

The most efficient way to work these muscles is to do a Super Kegel. It's best to do this exercise when your bladder is empty. You can do this exercise sitting or standing. Tighten the identified muscles and concentrate on keeping them as tight as possible. After a few seconds, you'll feel them begin to release. Renew your efforts to keep them as tight as possible. While you're working the muscles, you should feel tension or a mild tingling deep inside your body. If you don't, concentrate on tightening the muscles even more. Keep repeating the retightening for 20 seconds or the count of twenty. Do five of these Super Kegels a day, but don't do them all at once.

Because you know which muscles to tighten, you can consciously tighten them when you're about to sneeze, cough, or laugh. This and regularly emptying your bladder will help minimize any leakage.

Q ARE KEGELS JUST FOR PREGNANCY?

A Not at all. They're part of the postpartum exercise routine and can be started right after giving birth. (See pages 134–136 for more on postpartum comfort.) They're also part of a lifetime health routine that can prevent urinary incontinence.

LEG CRAMPS

Q SOME NIGHTS I WAKE UP WITH AN UNBEARABLE CRAMP IN MY CALF. HOW CAN I PREVENT THIS?

A Unfortunately, leg cramps are fairly common, especially late in pregnancy. Because a calcium-phosphorus imbalance may make cramps more likely, make sure to get the calcium you need and limit processed snack foods and soft drinks. Exercise seems to help. Try to walk a bit every day. Swimming is another good exercise.

Some care providers suggest working the calf muscles every day to improve circulation. This involves doing a foot pump. Women who already have cramping should just point their heel and then relax the stretch, repeating that ten times. Women who have not yet had leg cramps can first stretch their calf by pointing their heel, and then point their toes. Repeat this for ten heel-toe cycles for each foot.

You can also do a calf stretch (runner's stretch) by standing facing a wall a little less than an arm's length away. Put your palms on the wall and lean forward, bending your elbows and keeping your heels on the floor. You'll feel a stretch in your calf muscles. Hold that position for a count of five, then return to a standing position. Repeat for ten cycles.

When you go to bed, try to keep your legs warm. Cold may increase cramping. When stretching, avoid pointing your toes. If you do get a cramp, focus on pointing your heel. Your partner can help by gently pushing your toes toward your body. If you can get out of bed, a runner's stretch will help lengthen the cramping muscle.

SCREENING TESTS

Q WHAT IS A SCREENING TEST?

A Rather than giving everyone an expensive or complicated diagnostic test to determine if there's a problem, screening tests determine who is *most likely* to have a problem. This is a definite advantage because screening tests are quicker and easier than diagnostic tests. However, it can be an anxious time between getting a worrisome result from a screening test and the results of the diagnostic test. Two of the most common screening tests in pregnancy are the triple screen (or multiple marker) for birth defects and the glucose screening for gestational diabetes.

Q CAN I REFUSE A SCREENING TEST?

A You have the right to refuse any test or treatment. However, before you do, it's best to discuss your views with your care provider. At that time you can ask:
- How accurate is the screening test?
- What percentage of people actually have the condition when the screen is positive?
- How often does the screen miss people who have the condition?
- How long does it take to get the results?
- What happens if the screen is positive?
- What does the diagnostic test involve?
- How long does it take to get those results?
- How will a positive result affect my care?
- What decisions will I have to make if the results are positive?
- What happens if the test is negative, indicating I (or my baby) don't have the condition?
- Is there another way to get the information you're looking for?

ULTRASOUND

Q WHEN CAN I HAVE MY FIRST ULTRASOUND?

A Most expectant parents think of an ultrasound as a way to "see" their baby. However, it's best to use it as a screening or diagnostic tool.

Some care providers routinely schedule one or two ultrasounds during a pregnancy. Ask your provider what to expect.

Q WHAT ARE SOME REASONS TO HAVE AN ULTRASOUND?

A A diagnostic ultrasound or sonogram uses the echoes of high-frequency sound waves to produce an image. This image can be enhanced and recorded on a photograph, videotape, or DVD. The sound waves are sent and received by a transducer. Depending on the view needed, the transducer can be rubbed over the mother's abdomen or placed in her vagina. The procedure itself is not uncomfortable. However, in early pregnancy the woman needs to have a full bladder when having an abdominal ultrasound.

In early pregnancy an ultrasound is most often used:
• To make sure the embryo is in the uterus;
• To date the pregnancy;
• To determine the number of babies.

Ultrasound can also be used:
• To estimate the baby's growth;
• To make sure the baby is developing properly;
• To evaluate the position and condition of the placenta;
• To determine the position of the baby for amniocentesis or other procedures;
• To determine the baby's sex after the baby's genitals are visible.

Toward the end of pregnancy ultrasound can be used:
• To check the well-being of the baby;
• To determine the amount of amniotic fluid;
• To determine changes in the cervix;
• To verify the position of the baby and umbilical cord just before delivery.

Q A NEARBY BUSINESS OFFERS KEEPSAKE ULTRASOUNDS. IS THERE ANY REASON NOT TO TAKE ADVANTAGE OF THIS SERVICE?

A Diagnostic ultrasounds are considered safe. The studies on their safety were done at medical sites using trained personnel. Businesses offering keepsake sonograms are usually very clear that they are *not* diagnostic. Rather, they're done to provide video pictures or DVDs for expectant parents. Many care providers discourage women from having these scans because the businesses are not regulated. As a result, the equipment may not be precisely calibrated and the person doing the scan may not be adequately trained. In addition, there's a very small chance that the scan could show what appears to be a problem. This could be very upsetting until a diagnostic scan rules out the problem. If you want to get the scan for reassurance, talk to your care provider about your fears and concerns.

MULTIPLE MARKER/TRIPLE SCREEN

Q WHAT IS THE PURPOSE OF THE MULTIPLE MARKER TEST?

A The multiple marker is a blood test that screens for birth defects such as Down syndrome (a chromosomal defect that results in mental retardation), neural tube defects (such as spina bifida), and some other less common problems. The test is known by several names including *triple screen* and *maternal serum AFP*. It's done at 15–20 weeks.

This screen has a lot of false positive results, which means that most follow-up tests show the baby is healthy. Carrying more than one baby and incorrect dating of the pregnancy affect the result. If more testing is needed, an ultrasound is usually ordered. In addition, amniocentesis can determine if there's a chromosomal disorder or neural tube problem.

Some providers are using high-definition ultrasound rather than the multiple marker test. Talk with your care provider about your options.

CHORIONIC VILLUS SAMPLING (CVS) AND AMNIOCENTESIS

Q IS THERE A TEST THAT CAN BE DONE EARLY IN PREGNANCY TO DETERMINE IF THE BABY'S CHROMOSOMES ARE ALL RIGHT?

A Chorionic villus sampling (CVS) can be done as early as 10 weeks. This procedure uses a thin needle or catheter to remove a tiny amount of placental tissue. Because the placenta and baby have the same genetic makeup, this tissue can be analyzed for chromosomal problems. It usually takes about two weeks to get the results. The test cannot detect structural problems like neural tube defects.

The procedure increases the risk of miscarriage by about 1 percent. There's also a small risk of bleeding and infection. Because skill level affects the rate of test-related problems, it's best to use a center that's experienced at doing CVS. This test can be a good option when there's a risk of serious problems and there's a concern about continuing the pregnancy.

Q WHY IS AMNIOCENTESIS DONE?

A Amniocentesis is done to get information about the baby's condition. The procedure involves the removal of a small amount of amniotic fluid. Cells that are shed from the baby into the amniotic fluid are analyzed to determine if there's a chromosomal or genetic problem.

The amniotic fluid also contains hormones. Some of these indicate other kinds of birth defects such as neural tube problems. Amniocentesis is usually done between the 15th and 20th week. It takes about two weeks to get the test results.

In the third trimester amniocentesis can be done to determine the severity of blood disorders, such as Rh disease, and whether the baby's lungs have matured. The results from these tests come back quickly.

Q HOW IS AMNIOCENTESIS DONE?

A A long, thin needle is passed through the mother's abdomen and uterus into the amniotic sac. The physician uses ultrasound to determine exactly where to put the needle. There is less than a 1 percent chance that the procedure will cause a miscarriage or start labor. There is also a small risk of bleeding and infection.

GLUCOSE SCREENING

Q WHY DOES MY CARE PROVIDER WANT ME TO HAVE A GLUCOSE SCREENING WHEN I HAVEN'T GAINED EXCESSIVE WEIGHT?

A Care providers routinely order glucose screenings between the 24th and 28th week. This corresponds with the time the placenta starts creating a hormone that can result in the woman's blood sugar being too high. If this screening test is positive, a diagnostic test is done. The glucose tolerance test determines whether a woman has gestational diabetes. Women who have had gestational diabetes with a previous pregnancy are usually screened at the first prenatal visit. (See pages 73–74 for more on gestational diabetes.)

NON-STRESS TEST AND CONTRACTION STRESS TEST (CST)

Q WHAT'S THE DIFFERENCE BETWEEN A NON-STRESS TEST AND A CONTRACTION STRESS TEST?

A Toward the end of pregnancy it may be necessary to check on the baby's well-being. This is especially true if there's concern that the placenta is not able to deliver all the oxygen and nutrients the baby needs.

A non-stress test is relatively simple and can be done in the care provider's office. An electronic fetal monitor is placed on the mother's abdomen to continuously record the baby's heart rate. The baby is monitored for 20–30 minutes. During this time the mother indicates when she feels the baby move. The baby's heart rate should vary in response to movement. Sometimes sound or vibration is sent through the mother's abdomen to see how the baby's heart responds. A reactive heart rate indicates that the baby is doing well. If there isn't a lot of change, the care provider may order a contraction stress test.

A contraction stress test (CST), or oxytocin challenge test (OCT), is used in the last weeks of pregnancy to decide if labor should be induced or if a cesarean is needed. It's done in the hospital. This test also uses an electronic fetal monitor to track the baby's heart rate and the mother's uterine contractions. These contractions are induced, often by the drug Pitocin given through an IV. If the baby's heart rate responds normally to the contractions, the test is considered reassuring of the baby's well-being. A non-reassuring pattern indicates that the baby is not getting enough oxygen to handle the contractions well. This leads to a decision about whether labor should be induced or the baby should be born by cesarean.

BIOPHYSICAL PROFILE

Q I'M SCHEDULED FOR A BIOPHYSICAL PROFILE. IS THAT SERIOUS?

A A biophysical profile is a way to determine how well the baby is doing in the last weeks of pregnancy. The tests are not uncomfortable and the profile gives a comprehensive picture of the baby's status.

The profile has five components. First, an ultrasound is used to determine the amount of amniotic fluid. Too much or very little amniotic fluid indicates a problem. A normal amount indicates the baby's kidneys and the placenta are working well. Next, the ultrasound is used to analyze the baby's muscle tone, movements, and breathing motions. Lastly, a non-stress test is used to assess the responsiveness of the baby's heart rate.

There are also variations of the profile. One common variation is a non-stress test and an ultrasound to determine the amount of amniotic fluid.

HYPEREMESIS GRAVIDARUM

Q I'M 12 WEEKS PREGNANT AND STILL HAVE SEVERE NAUSEA AND VOMITING. WHAT'S WRONG?

A Severe nausea and vomiting is exhausting as well as disruptive. If you're finding it difficult to function, contact your care provider. There are prescription medicines that can help. In addition, some women have found complementary therapies like acupuncture effective. Staying on top of the nausea will help you feel better and resume daily activities, including more normal eating.

Less than 2 percent of women have such serious problems with vomiting that they need medical treatment. The biggest concern is dehydration because it can put both the mother's and baby's health at risk. Therefore, concentrate on drinking a lot of fluid. If you become dehydrated, you may need fluids through an IV. For most women, the hyperemesis eases by the 16th week. (See page 6 for tips on coping with morning sickness.)

Warning Signs

Call your care provider if you have:
- A fever over 101°F;
- Severe or persistent vomiting or diarrhea;
- Pain, burning, or trouble with urination;
- Unusual vaginal discharge or bleeding;
- Unusual or severe cramping or abdominal pain;
- Severe headaches;
- Fainting spells or persistent dizziness;
- Blurred vision or spots before your eyes;
- Swelling in your hands, fingers, or face;
- Difficulty breathing or shortness of breath that seems to be getting worse;
- Signs of preterm labor (See page 123.);
- After 28 weeks, noticeable changes in your baby's movement;
- A strong feeling that something isn't right.

GESTATIONAL DIABETES

Q MY GLUCOSE TOLERANCE TEST INDICATES THAT I HAVE GESTATIONAL DIABETES. WHAT DOES THAT MEAN?

A It means that the level of glucose (sugar) in your blood is too high. Blood sugar is controlled by insulin. During pregnancy the placenta produces a hormone to reduce the effect of insulin. This makes more sugar available to the growing baby. In some women too much sugar stays in the blood. That can result in the baby growing too large or in problems with the placenta. In addition, if your blood sugar is not well controlled during pregnancy, the baby may have serious problems with her own sugar balance after birth. Early detection of a high blood sugar level means the condition can be treated before complications develop.

Most likely you'll need to monitor your blood sugar level until the baby is born. Dietary changes and moderate exercise may be enough to keep your blood sugar under control. Sometimes insulin injections are necessary. Your blood sugar level will likely return to normal after your baby is born. However, women who develop gestational diabetes are at risk for developing diabetes later in life.

PREGNANCY-INDUCED HYPERTENSION (PIH) AND PREECLAMPSIA

Q WHAT IS PIH?

A PIH refers to the condition in which an expectant woman's blood pressure is high after the 20th week of pregnancy. If the blood pressure is not controlled, it will create problems for the baby and mother. High blood pressure can damage the placenta and endanger the baby's oxygen and nutrient supply. High blood pressure can also damage the mother's circulatory system, liver, and kidneys. Severe PIH can threaten the life of the mother and her baby.

Q WHAT IS PREECLAMPSIA?

A Preeclampsia used to be called toxemia. The symptoms are high blood pressure, protein in the urine, and edema (swelling). The swelling involves the hands and face as well as the feet and ankles. As the condition gets worse, a woman may have a bad headache, dizziness, visual disturbances, and pain very high in her abdomen. Several of the procedures done at prenatal visits, including checking weight, urine, and blood pressure, are aimed at detecting preeclampsia. If not controlled, this condition can lead to very serious problems including eclampsia (maternal seizures) and HELLP syndrome. (HELLP is a complication that can damage a woman's blood vessels, nervous system, and organs as well as endanger her developing baby.)

Q WHY IS BED REST ORDERED WHEN A WOMAN HAS SIGNS OF PREECLAMPSIA?

A Being put on bed rest at home is often the first step in treating early preeclampsia. The woman spends most of her time lying on her side. The side-lying position lowers blood pressure and improves circulation to the uterus and placenta.

It's important that a woman follow her care provider's instructions. If resting at home does not improve her condition, she may need to be hospitalized. Medication may also be needed to prevent further complications. Occasionally, it's necessary to deliver the baby early. Usually the mother's blood pressure returns to normal soon after giving birth.

RH NEGATIVE

Q I'M RH NEGATIVE AND MY PARTNER IS RH POSITIVE. DOES THAT MEAN I'LL HAVE TO HAVE SPECIAL CARE DURING MY PREGNANCY?

A Rh is a blood factor. People who have this factor are Rh positive. Those who don't are Rh negative. Women who are Rh positive don't have to worry about the Rh factor. When a woman is Rh negative and the father of the baby is Rh positive, the baby may be Rh positive or Rh negative. If the baby is Rh negative, there's no problem. If the baby is Rh positive, the woman's body may make antibodies that destroy her baby's blood, causing the baby to be anemic.

Because it takes exposure to Rh positive blood to start the antibody process, first babies are usually not at risk. One of the blood tests done at the first or second prenatal visit looks for Rh antibodies. If that test shows there are no antibodies, you don't have to worry. Most likely you'll get a shot of Rh immune globulin (Rhogam) at 28 weeks. Rhogam temporarily prevents your body from making antibodies. In addition, you'll get Rhogam after invasive procedures, like chorionic villus sampling (CVS) and amniocentesis, or uterine bleeding. Then, after your baby is born, you'll get another shot if your baby is Rh positive. This is done to protect future pregnancies.

If your blood shows antibodies and your baby is Rh positive, you'll be frequently monitored. Your baby may need a blood transfusion after birth if the anemia is serious. If necessary, a perinatal center can give your baby a transfusion while your baby is still in the womb.

Ask your care provider to explain your antibody status and what will be done to care for this baby and to protect future pregnancies.

TWINS

Q MY ULTRASOUND CONFIRMED THAT I'M CARRYING TWINS. HOW WILL THAT CHANGE WHAT I CAN DO?

A A multiple pregnancy (carrying more than one baby) puts additional stress on a mother's body and can increase pregnancy discomforts. It's very important to take good care of yourself. However, check with your care provider before taking any over-the-counter or home remedies for discomforts. In addition, make sure you eat well. That means eating foods high in protein, iron, and calcium and getting more than the additional 300 calories per day. Your care provider will help you determine your healthy weight gain and calorie intake. If you're finding it difficult to get all the nutrients you need, ask for a consultation with a nutritionist.

Because your body is working hard to grow two babies, it's important to have a rest each day. You may also need to start cutting back on activities, including vigorous exercise. Consider getting help with household chores and passing up social responsibilities. You may have to stop working sooner than you had planned. Toward the end of pregnancy, you may be put on bed rest.

Because twins are at risk of being born prematurely, you'll have more than the usual number of prenatal visits. This monitoring of your health and your babies' development is designed to help you carry the pregnancy to 37 weeks. Then, your babies will be mature enough not to need special care after birth.

Finding out that you're carrying twins can be both exciting and over-whelming. Consider getting information and support from other families with twins. Ask your provider to give you the number of a local support group, or visit www.nomotc.org.

OVER AGE 35

Q I'M OVER 35 AND THIS IS MY FIRST BABY. DOES THAT MAKE MY PREGNANCY HIGH RISK?

A Although many care providers use that label, it may be better to define your pregnancy as being at higher risk for certain conditions. Although age may increase wisdom, it also increases the likelihood of medical conditions such as heart disease, diabetes, and fibroids. Older pregnant women are more likely to develop pregnancy-induced hypertension (PIH) and gestational diabetes, especially if they're overweight before pregnancy. In addition, there's an increased risk of the baby having a chromosomal problem like Down syndrome. The older a woman is, the greater the risk. Although your age puts you at greater risk, it doesn't mean you'll have any of these problems. Most women over the age of 35 have healthy pregnancies and healthy babies.

There are some things you can do to maximize the chances of having a healthy pregnancy. Living as healthy a lifestyle as you can will help your body grow a healthy baby. This includes eating well, keeping your weight gain to the recommended amount, and not smoking or drinking alcohol. Because older mothers are at risk for preterm labor, try to reduce the amount of stress in your life. This may include limiting activities and responsibilities at home and at work so you can get the rest you need.

Keeping all your prenatal appointments is also very important. That way your care provider can monitor your health and respond if there's a problem.

MISCARRIAGE

Q**WHAT CAN I DO TO PREVENT A MISCARRIAGE?**

A Miscarriage is the loss of a developing baby before 20 weeks. It's rarely the result of something the mother did. Most miscarriages happen because of a chromosomal problem, infection, or a problem with the placenta. Although you may not be able to prevent a miscarriage, you can focus on having a healthy pregnancy. (See pages 14–31.)

A woman who has had a miscarriage should ask her care provider if there are any health issues she should address before the next pregnancy. She can also get the provider's recommendation about how long to wait before trying to get pregnant. Most women who have a miscarriage go on to have a healthy pregnancy.

Q**I FELL YESTERDAY AND NOW I'M WORRIED THAT I'LL LOSE THE PREGNANCY.**

A Although novels and movies often depict a woman's pregnancy ending after she falls, this is rarely the case in reality. Major trauma or a severe blow to the abdomen can affect a pregnancy, but a simple fall usually does not. See the warning signs at left for things to watch for. Also, contact your care provider so you can get more reassurance.

Signs of a Possible Miscarriage

Call your care provider if you experience:
- Pain in your abdomen for more than a day;
- Bleeding that's like a period;
- Both bleeding and cramping;
- Pain that's been growing stronger over the past two hours.

If you're unable to talk with your care provider immediately, seek help from Emergency Services if you experience:
- Vaginal bleeding that soaks more than two sanitary pads in an hour;
- Bleeding that contains clots or other matter;
- Severe pain.

Q MY FRIEND HAD A MISCARRIAGE RIGHT AFTER I GOT PREGNANT, AND I FEEL A LITTLE GUILTY BEING PREGNANT WHEN SHE ISN'T. IS THERE ANYTHING I CAN DO?

A The loss of a developing baby, even early in the pregnancy, can be a shock, even a devastating loss. Each person deals with miscarriage in his or her own way. The grieving time varies. However, most parents say that support from family and friends is extremely helpful. You can share your feelings with your friend and find out what she would like you to do. Then you can interact with her in a way you know is helpful.

HAVING A SECOND (OR LATER) BABY

Q I'VE ALREADY HAD A BABY. HOW DOES THAT AFFECT THIS PREGNANCY?

A Women having their first baby are PREGNANT. Multips (women having their second or later baby) are pregnant. That is, they tend to be less caught up in the process because they're familiar with the physical changes. For example, although multips feel the signs of pregnancy earlier, these may not seem as remarkable or distressing. However, if a woman's previous pregnancy was difficult, she may feel anxious about the condition recurring. Make sure to share any concerns you have with your care provider. That way he or she can either assure you that things are going well or can help you address the issue.

You may be surprised by how much work it is to be pregnant. This can be magnified if you're extremely busy balancing work, home, and the needs of an older child or children. If it's been more than a couple of years since your first or previous baby was born, you may feel you have less energy than before.

Multips spend less time daydreaming about the baby and more time worrying about how the older child or children will respond. You will be more focused on integrating your new baby into the household.

There are some specific differences in how your body responds to pregnancy. You'll look pregnant sooner and will be more likely to carry the baby lower due to decreased abdominal muscle tone. You'll also feel the baby move about a month earlier than last time. That's because in addition to decreased muscle tone, you'll know what these movements feel like.

In the end you'll probably feel that this pregnancy is a lot like, yet different from, your last one. That's because each pregnancy is unique.

SECTION TWO
Childbirth

HOW LABOR WORKS

Q WHAT IS LABOR?

A Labor is the work a woman's body does to birth a baby. Uterine contractions shorten and open the cervix then push the baby through the woman's vagina. After the baby is born, additional contractions birth the placenta.

Q WHY IS LABOR DIVIDED INTO STAGES?

A Labor is divided into stages to describe the process. During the first stage, the cervix thins and opens. This is the longest stage, lasting twelve hours or more for a first baby. The first stage is divided into phases that describe the process of dilation (opening). During the second stage, the baby is pushed through the vagina and is born. This can take several hours for a first baby. The third stage is the period after the baby is born until the placenta is delivered. This usually takes 10–20 minutes, sometimes a bit longer. Some providers refer to the first two hours after birth as the fourth stage. During this time the woman's body begins the recovery process.

THE UTERUS AND CERVIX

Q HOW CAN MY UTERUS GET SO BIG?

A The uterus is a muscular organ. For the first half of pregnancy, it grows by adding cells. Then, for the rest of pregnancy, these cells stretch. This enables the uterus to grow from the size of a pear to that of a small watermelon. What's equally amazing is that at about 6 weeks after birth, the uterus returns to nearly its original size.

Q WHY DO CARE PROVIDERS DO CERVICAL CHECKS?

A At the first prenatal visit a care provider checks the cervix for changes that indicate pregnancy. Later in pregnancy the cervix may be checked for changes that indicate labor is beginning. During labor, cervical checks monitor the dilation (opening) of the cervix.

The cervix is the opening from the uterus to the vagina. It's about an inch long and is located at the top of the vagina. You can feel it with your index finger. (If you want to gently check your cervix, it's best to wash your hands first.) When you aren't pregnant, your cervix feels firm, like the tip of your nose. During pregnancy your cervix gets softer and feels more like your earlobe. Just before going into labor your cervix gets even softer, like your lips. In labor it will be stretchy, like the inside of your cheek.

At the beginning of pregnancy, increased circulation gives the cervix a darker color. This change is one of the signs of pregnancy that a care provider checks for. Toward the end of pregnancy changes in the shape of the cervix indicate the woman is moving toward labor. Most of labor is devoted to opening the cervix so a baby can be born through the vagina.

Q WHY DOESN'T MY CARE PROVIDER CHECK MY CERVIX AT EVERY PRENATAL VISIT?

A At the first visit a care provider usually examines the cervix to make sure it's normal and does a Pap test to check for disease. After that, there normally isn't a need to check the cervix until about the last month of pregnancy. At those visits your care provider will be looking for signs of cervical change. If you begin having contractions that could indicate the beginning of preterm labor, your care provider will check to see if your cervix has begun to change. (See page 123 for more on preterm labor.)

Q HOW DOES THE CERVIX CHANGE? WHAT MAKES THAT HAPPEN?

A First, hormones ripen or soften the cervix. Then uterine contractions pull on the cervix causing it to shorten or get thinner (efface) and open (dilate). Effacement is usually expressed as a percentage. When the cervix is about half an inch long, it's said to be 50 percent effaced. Effacement makes it possible for the cervix to stretch and open. When the cervix is completely thinned, it's 100 percent effaced.

Dilation is measured in centimeters. During pregnancy the cervix stays closed. In late pregnancy it begins to thin. After that, it begins to open (dilate). At first it will dilate the width of a fingertip (about 1 cm). It will then gradually dilate until it is completely opened at 10 cm. The first time the cervix opens in labor, it's tight and does considerable thinning before it does a lot of dilating. If you've already experienced a labor that opened your cervix to at least 5 cm, your cervix will open more easily and do more effacing and dilating at the same time. This can make for a shorter labor.

Q WHAT'S THE PURPOSE OF THE MUCOUS PLUG?

A One of the changes of pregnancy is that the cervix secretes thick mucus that remains in the opening of the cervix, acting like a plug. It provides a physical barrier that helps protect the amniotic sac (the place where the baby grows). At the end of pregnancy, the cervix begins to change shape and the plug gets discharged through the vagina. You may find some of this mucus in your underwear or on a piece of toilet paper. After the plug is gone, the cervix secretes thinner mucus. Losing your mucous plug is a positive sign that indicates your cervix is changing shape. It's not necessarily a sign that labor has begun.

Q WHAT IS BLOODY SHOW?

A After the mucous plug is gone, the cervix secretes slippery mucus called "show." As the cervix thins and opens, small blood vessels break and tinge the mucus. This is called "bloody show" and is a sign of cervical change. Bloody show gets heavier as the first stage of labor progresses. Brown-tinged mucus indicates old blood, while red indicates fresh blood. Brown-tinged show can appear after a cervical exam or sex and is not a concern. If there's more blood than mucus, contact your care provider. This could be a sign of blood coming from someplace other than the cervix.

CONTRACTIONS

Q WHAT ARE BRAXTON-HICKS CONTRACTIONS?

A Braxton-Hicks contractions are your uterus exercising. They help maintain uterine muscle tone and improve blood flow. These contractions occur throughout pregnancy, although they're not usually felt until the second trimester. As your uterus gets larger, you'll feel them more frequently. Women who have already had a baby feel these contractions earlier and more often than first-time moms.

During Braxton-Hicks contractions the uterus gets hard, rather like making a fist. Then it relaxes and feels soft again. These contractions are not painful but can be uncomfortable, especially toward the end of pregnancy. Although they're not strong enough to do the work of labor, they do help the cervix get ready for labor. If you have five or more contractions in an hour, it may be a sign that you're in early labor. If this happens when you're less than 37 weeks, see page 123 for signs of preterm labor. If you're 37 weeks or more, see pages 88–90 for information about prodromal and false labor.

Q WHAT'S THE DIFFERENCE BETWEEN BRAXTON-HICKS CONTRACTIONS AND LABOR CONTRACTIONS?

A The bottom line is that Braxton-Hicks contractions do not cause significant cervical change, as labor contractions do. The two types also differ in intensity and coordination. Labor contractions are stronger because they involve the whole uterus, and the muscle cells work in a more coordinated way. Labor contractions start at the top of the uterus (called the fundus) and have the effect of pushing the baby down toward the cervix. These contractions also pull up on the cervix, causing it to thin out and open up.

Braxton-Hicks contractions tend to be felt mostly in the abdomen. Labor contractions may be felt in the front or the back. If they start in the back, they often sweep around the sides to the front. They also cause a feeling of vaginal fullness or pressure. Sometimes labor contractions are felt mostly in the back. (See page 90 for information on back labor.)

Q HOW DO YOU TIME CONTRACTIONS?

A Contractions are timed to determine two things: frequency and duration. To determine the frequency (how far apart they are), time from the beginning of one contraction to the beginning of the next. This time will be in minutes and will include both the contraction and the rest period until the next contraction. If you're at 38 weeks or later, don't bother to time contractions that are more than 10 minutes apart. If your contractions are more than 7 or 8 minutes apart, try to do other things in addition to timing the contractions. Usually the hard work of labor is done with contractions coming closer than 5 minutes apart.

To determine the duration of a contraction, time from when you feel the contraction start until you no longer feel it. At the beginning of labor, contractions are likely to increase in intensity for 15–30 seconds and then let up. Once labor is well established, contractions commonly last about a minute. Sometimes they can last up to 90 seconds.

THE BABY'S POSITION

Q YESTERDAY THE SHAPE OF MY BELLY CHANGED. I'VE HEARD ABOUT BABIES DROPPING. IS THAT WHAT HAPPENED?

A Up until now your baby has been able to easily change positions in the womb. Yesterday the baby's head settled into your pelvis. This is called lightening because the weight of the pregnancy seems to lighten. It will be a bit easier for you to breathe, and you may have less heartburn. On the other hand, you'll probably need to urinate more frequently because your baby's head is closer to your bladder.

At your next visit your care provider can do a vaginal exam to confirm that your baby's head has settled into the pelvis and is engaged. Engagement means the top of the head is at 0 station. (See below.) For first pregnancies, engagement commonly occurs before labor starts. Women who have already had a baby may find that engagement occurs during labor.

Q WHAT DOES *STATION* MEAN?

A Station describes where the baby's presenting part is located within the mother's pelvis. The presenting part is the part of the baby coming out first. Usually that's the top of the baby's head. Zero station is the middle of the pelvis at the ischial spines. Negative numbers indicate the head (or presenting part) is above these bones. If the head is at –4, it's above the level of the pubic bone. At 0 the head is engaged in the pelvis. Positive numbers indicate the head is below the ischial spines and moving toward birth. The lowest station is +5 and means the head is being born.

Q HOW IMPORTANT IS IT THAT THE BABY BE HEAD DOWN FOR BIRTH?

A About 95 percent of the time, the baby's head is the presenting part. This is the best presentation for a vaginal birth. When the buttocks or feet are the presenting part, the baby is in a breech position. Care providers most often deliver a breech baby by cesarean. If the shoulder is the presenting part, the baby will be born by cesarean if the presentation persists.

Q MY FRIEND HAD A LONG LABOR BECAUSE HER BABY WAS
IN THE POSTERIOR POSITION. WHAT DOES THAT MEAN?

A Another factor in labor is position. It describes the way the baby is
facing. The term refers specifically to the position of the presenting
part. When it's the head, the reference point is the back of the baby's head.
During labor the position changes as the head rotates through the pelvis.
Because the top (or inlet) of the pelvis is wider side-to-side, the head enters
so that the baby is facing the mother's side. The bottom (or outlet) of the
pelvis is wider front-to-back. That means the head has to turn in order to fit
through. Usually the best way is for the back of the baby's head to rotate
toward the mother's front (anterior). If the baby rotates so the back of the
baby's head is toward the mother's back, the position is called posterior. To
visualize your baby's position, imagine lying on your back. In the anterior
position your baby would be looking at the floor. In the posterior position
your baby would be looking at the ceiling.
  Many babies who start out posterior rotate to anterior in order to fit
through the pelvis. This takes time. Sometimes the baby can fit through in
the posterior position, but the descent takes longer. Some babies whose
heads are in the posterior position need to be born by cesarean because
labor stops progressing.

RESPONDING TO LABOR

Q HOW SOON SHOULD I CALL MY CARE PROVIDER WHEN
I THINK MY LABOR IS BEGINNING?

A Care providers usually have a set of instructions for what to do when
labor starts. You may be asked to call the office during office hours
and a night number after hours. Some providers have you call the birth
facility first. Follow these instructions. In addition, you can call either your
provider or the facility if you have questions or are worried. Make sure to
call immediately if you start bleeding or leaking fluid from your vagina.

Q WHAT SHOULD I DO IF MY BAG OF WATERS BREAKS?

A Your baby has been floating in amniotic fluid in the amniotic sac. (See
pages 54–55.) This sac, also called the membranes, can get a tear and

leak fluid. About one in six labors starts this way. Notify your care provider according to the instructions you were given. Your care provider will want to know:

- If you're having contractions now;
- What time your membranes broke or started leaking;
- Whether this started with a gush or just dampness;
- What the fluid looks like. Amniotic fluid looks clear. Fluid that is dark, greenish, or streaked with black or dark green indicates that the baby has had a bowel movement. Sometimes this happens when the baby has been stressed.
- What the fluid smells like. Amniotic fluid has a slightly sweet smell, although you may not be able to detect any odor. Fluid that smells "bad" may indicate an infection.

This information will enable your care provider to determine how quickly you should leave for the hospital or birth center. Once your membranes break, you'll leak fluid with each contraction and with abdominal pressure from a cough or laugh. Use a sanitary napkin or towel to absorb the fluid. DO NOT insert a tampon or put anything into your vagina.

Q WHAT IF I CAN'T TELL IF I'M LEAKING FLUID OR URINE?

A If you have constant dampness and you're not sure whether you're leaking amniotic fluid, call your care provider's office or the birth facility. You can have the fluid tested to determine whether it's amniotic fluid.

KINDS OF LABOR

Q WHAT IS FALSE LABOR?

A When a woman has contractions over several hours but experiences no cervical change, it's called false labor. Many women have bouts of contractions before they go into labor. If you've already had a baby, you're more likely to have contractions that start and stop.

There are some things you can do to help you determine if you're in labor. (See the box on page 89.) Remember, if you're not at least 37 weeks, call your care provider if you begin to have contractions or a backache that comes and goes with a regular pattern (six per hour) or if you think your bag of waters may be leaking.

Q WHAT IS PRODROMAL LABOR?

A Prodromal labor is very early labor. Many times a woman's body eases into labor, moving the cervix forward so it's in the best position for labor and thinning it out so it can open. Rather than happening over several hours, this takes place over days or a week or more. It can be frustrating and tiring to have contractions that start and stop. However, any work done before your "labor day" is work that doesn't have to be done during labor.

Q I'VE BEEN IN PRODRO-MAL LABOR FOR SEV-ERAL NIGHTS AND I'M NOT SLEEPING. I'M AFRAID I'LL BE TOO EXHAUSTED TO GO THROUGH LABOR. WHAT CAN I DO?

A Check with your care provider. Your options will depend on your due date and the amount of cervical change. If the decision is to wait and let things unfold:

- Try some of the sleep suggestions on page 44.
- Take a warm bath. This can temporarily reduce the blood concentration of oxytocin (the hormone that stimulates contractions) and may give you time for a good post-bath nap.
- Take time during the day to rest.
- Make sure you're eating well and drinking plenty of fluids. Skipping meals can increase your sense of fatigue.

Distinguishing between False Labor and Effective Labor Contractions

- *Are they regular?* Most of the time labor contractions have a rhythm and get closer together over time. False labor contractions may be irregular, even erratic. If they're regular, they won't have the other characteristics of an effective labor contraction.
- *Are they getting longer?* Labor contractions usually last at least a minute. If they start out shorter than 60 seconds, they get longer over time.
- *Are they getting stronger?* Sometimes this can be hard to determine because anxiety, fatigue, and a full bladder can make contractions feel stronger. Effective labor contractions often feel like a lot of vaginal pressure and may include a backache. At the least, the contractions shouldn't feel like they're decreasing in intensity.
- *Does changing my activity cause the contractions to decrease?* If you've been sitting or walking, try lying down. If you've been lying down, get up and walk around. If the change in activity results in a decrease in uterine activity, this means the contractions are not yet effective labor contractions.

- Try not to anticipate the next contraction. When your labor gets organized, the changed quality of the contractions will alert you to the need to pay closer attention.

Q WHAT IS BACK LABOR?

A This is the term used for labor contractions that are felt mostly in the back. The baby may be positioned so that the back of the baby's head is toward the mother's spine. Every contraction may cause a severe backache that decreases between contractions but may not go away entirely. Pain relief is aimed at reducing the pain and helping the baby turn to a better position.

Counterpressure usually works best during contractions. This can include pressing on the woman's back using hands or round objects like tennis balls or a rolling pin. Using a cold compress may also be helpful. Wrap the ice or frozen object in a towel to prevent damaging the woman's skin. A soft blue-ice pack or a frozen juice can are convenient options.

Between contractions warmth and gentle massage may be comforting. Try a hot water bottle or rice sock warmed in the microwave. Again, remember to protect the woman's skin by wrapping the object in a towel. Laboring in the shower and directing the spray toward the lower back may also decrease back pain.

The mother's position and movement can help the baby turn to a better position. Positions that use gravity involve being on hands and knees or lying over a birth ball. A side-lying position with the upper knee bent and brought close to the chest may help the baby rotate. Pelvic rocking can both comfort the mother and help the baby move. Walking and stair climbing are other activities to try.

EARLY LABOR

Q WHAT DOES IT FEEL LIKE WHEN LABOR BEGINS?

A Often labor begins with contractions that feel like cramps, a backache, or a lot of pelvic pressure. These contractions may bring a mix of emotions. You may be surprised or relieved that labor has started. At the same time you may feel anxious about dealing with the contractions. This can be especially true if the first contractions are stronger than you expected. It's helpful to have someone you can call to give you reassurance, such as a doula. (See pages 115–118.) She can provide some perspective and suggest ways to stay as comfortable as possible.

Early Labor Checklist

- Get the telephone numbers of your care provider and birth facility, and put them by the phone.
- If it's nighttime, try to get more rest. If you can't sleep, lie as comfortably as you can. Do whatever is soothing or comforting:
  * Dim the lights.
  * Listen to soft music.
  * Try aromatherapy.
  * Get a back rub or foot massage from your partner.
  * Do some gentle stretches while taking a warm shower. Follow this with some relaxation breathing. (See pages 59–60.)
  If you feel a need to be up and active, use upright positions and movement to stimulate early labor:
  * Walk around.
  * Rock in a rocking chair.
  * Sit on an exercise or birth ball.
  * Try alternating activity and rest.
- If it's daytime and you're tired, try to get some more rest. (See the suggestions above.) If you're restless and have a lot of nervous energy, alternate nonstrenuous activity with something that can distract your attention:
  * Play a board game or card game.
  * Watch TV or a video.
  * Go to a movie.
  * Make or bake something you can eat as part of the birth celebration.
- Are you hungry? When did you eat last? Labor requires a lot of energy. It's important to maintain fluids and eat lightly, as if you had an upset stomach. Many cultures encourage giving laboring women sweetened tea to drink.
- Do your labor support people know you may need them soon? If your partner isn't with you, contact him or her. Call the person who will provide additional labor support. If you have other children, notify whoever will be taking care of them.
- Are the items you want to bring to the hospital or birth center packed and ready to go?

Q HOW LONG DOES EARLY LABOR LAST?

A Early labor is usually the longest phase of the first stage. There's a lot of variation in how long it takes for the cervix to open to 4–5 cm. Some women begin by having prodromal labor over several days or a week. (See pages 89–90.) Others start with strong contractions that accomplish this dilation in a matter of hours.

During this early phase of labor you can usually walk and talk through your contractions. If the contraction makes you stop what you're doing, you can return to your activity right after the contraction ends. The coping strategies for early labor include things that help you pass the time. (See the box on page 91.)

Q WHEN SHOULD I GO TO THE HOSPITAL?

A Unless there's a special circumstance, like your bag of waters has broken or your care provider has given you special instructions, the decision is mostly yours. It's usually more comfortable to stay home in early labor. There are more options for passing the time until the contractions get stronger. It's also easier to be up and moving around, which may help stimulate labor.

Many women plan on going to the hospital or birth center when their contractions get more intense. The fact that you want to go to the hospital doesn't mean that birth is imminent. If at any time you feel anxious about staying home, call your provider or the birth facility.

Q MY FRIEND WENT TO THE HOSPITAL WITH STRONG CONTRACTIONS BUT WAS SENT HOME. WHY DID THIS HAPPEN?

A Some providers prefer that labor be well established before admitting a woman. This requires checking cervical dilation. If the exam indicates that the labor is still in the early phase, a woman may be advised to go home for a while. If this happens to you, ask as many questions as needed to understand what kind of change the staff is looking for. In addition, ask what you can do—and what you should avoid—while you're waiting to return. If you're worried about leaving the hospital, share your concerns. That way you can make a plan that you're comfortable with.

Q MY PARTNER IS VERY WORRIED THAT WE WON'T GET TO THE HOSPITAL IN TIME.

A Many partners worry about this. TV and movies often show childbirth as sudden or filled with unexpected events. Your partner probably feels you'll be safest in the hospital where professionals will know what to do. Because it's his or her responsibility to get you there, your partner may feel the earlier this happens the better. A doula can be very helpful to a labor partner. She can provide reassurance and help you think through any decision you have to make. (See pages 115–118.)

One thing your partner can do ahead of time is figure out several routes to the hospital. That way, if there's construction or a traffic jam, you'll know alternate routes. It's also a good idea to keep the gas tank at least half full so you don't have to worry about running out of gas.

ACTIVE LABOR

Q HOW LONG DOES IT TAKE TO GET FROM 5 CM TO FULL DILATION?

A The length of time it takes to get to 5 cm is not a predictor of the time it will take for complete dilation. After the cervix gets to 4–5 cm, the rate of dilation usually increases to about 1 cm every one to two hours. However, the position of the baby can affect the rate. If the baby's head is not in the best position for birth, contractions work to turn the baby to a better position. This commonly happens when the back of the baby's head is toward the mother's spine. During that time there may be little progress in dilation.

Q WHAT MAKES ACTIVE LABOR DIFFERENT FROM EARLY LABOR?

A Active labor is more intense. You and your body are getting quite serious about having this baby. In addition to being stronger, the contractions last longer and come closer together. You'll want to focus on working with the contraction and then resting until the next one. Many women don't feel like chatting between contractions, and some find the conversation of others annoying, especially during a contraction. Your choice of comfort measures and way of coping with active labor will be unique to you. (See pages 100–106.)

Q WHAT HAPPENS IN TRANSITION?

A Transition is the term used for the last few centimeters of dilation when contractions are at their greatest intensity. They can last up to 90 seconds and be 2–3 minutes apart. That leaves little time to rest between contractions. You may also have physical signs that your body is working very hard, such as trembling or vomiting. Although transition is intense, it's relatively short. It may be less than an hour.

Labor Partner's Checklist during Active Labor

- *Am I physically comfortable?* Labor partners can end up in positions that may strain their backs or joints. Consider sitting in a chair rather than leaning over the bed to maintain eye contact with the laboring woman. Also, try bracing against a wall or sitting behind her if you're supporting her weight.
- *Do I need a break?* Try to take a break before she gets to 7 cm. After that you may not get a chance. If there isn't an additional support person, ask the nurse to stay in the room while you take a break. Take the time to use the bathroom, do some stretches, or just get outside the room for a few minutes if you're feeling overwhelmed.
- *When did I last eat?* Make sure to eat and drink regularly. Low blood sugar can make you feel faint or dizzy.
- *Am I asking simple yes-or-no questions to make sure that what I'm doing is what she needs?* As labor progresses, her needs will change. Ask her, "Is my (technique) helping?" or "Do you want me to continue (action)?" If the answer is no, remember that she's rejecting the technique, not you. She still needs your support.

SECOND STAGE

Q DOES THE URGE TO PUSH INDICATE THAT LABOR HAS REACHED THE SECOND STAGE?

A The need to bear down or push is part of the second stage. However, the baby's position can stimulate an urge to push even though the cervix isn't fully opened. Sometimes the cervix is almost fully dilated except for a small lip. This is why you're not supposed to push until your cervix has been checked. Pushing before the cervix is fully opened can cause it to swell, slowing labor progress. If the urge is premature, you'll probably be told to pant lightly or blow out to prevent holding your breath and bearing down.

It's also possible for your cervix to be fully dilated and for your baby's head to have entered the vagina, yet you don't feel an urge to push. Your body is resting during this pause. After this rest the urge to push will begin to grow in intensity. Waiting until you have a definite urge to push makes your efforts more effective.

If you've had an epidural or spinal anesthetic, you may need to be coached on when to push because the medication can block these messages.

Q WHAT IS SPONTANEOUS PUSHING?

A If you can feel the urge to push and can move freely, many providers believe the best way to push is to follow your body's messages. During the contraction you alternate light breathing with periods of holding your breath and bearing down. You may or may not make a sound while pushing. This technique is the least stressful on your heart and blood vessels and is an effective way to add to the power of your uterus. Your nurse or care provider may encourage your pushing efforts but won't orchestrate your pushing. This spontaneous method may not be as fast as directed pushing, but it isn't as exhausting and seems to be easier on the baby.

Q WHAT IS DIRECTED PUSHING?

A If you don't feel the urge to push because of pain medication, or you're having difficulty working with the rhythm of your contractions, you may be directed when to push. Your nurse or caregiver will tell you when to start and stop bearing down. When the contraction begins, you'll take a couple of deep breaths and then hold your breath and bear down. Often the goal is to push for 5–7 seconds. (Longer breath-holding can be hard on your circulatory system and can reduce oxygen to the baby.) Then you'll be told to let out that breath, take another breath, and hold that one. Making sounds is usually discouraged. Your nurse, provider, and partner may keep urging you to push harder. This technique may also be used if a baby needs to be born faster than the pace of spontaneous pushing.

Q EXACTLY HOW DO YOU PUSH?

A Pushing in labor is most like making yourself pee faster. You can try this for a few seconds while you're urinating. Take in a breath and then bear down with your abdominal muscles. This should make the stream of urine come out harder and faster. Once you've done this, you really don't have to practice bearing down.

Sometimes early in the second stage it's hard to get the pushing force directed properly. If that happens, your nurse or care provider can put two fingers inside your vagina and press toward your rectum. Then you can concentrate on pushing those fingers out. After a few good pushes you probably won't need that assistance.

Q WHAT'S THE BEST POSITION FOR PUSHING?

A The best position depends on many factors including the position of the baby and how fast the baby is moving through the pelvis. A mother may prefer a particular position or need to be in a specific position for medical reasons. Care providers may also prefer a particular position. Talk to your provider ahead of time about preferred pushing positions.

Upright positions like squatting and sitting on a birth stool can make it easier for the baby to move down through the pelvis. Side-lying and being on hands and knees can help a baby get into a better position. Lying on the side or back can slow the progress of a baby coming too quickly.

Q HOW LONG DOES THE PUSHING USUALLY TAKE?

A It usually takes an hour and a half to two hours (or more) for a first baby, although some come more quickly. For women who've had a previous vaginal birth, the second (or later) baby usually comes faster than the first. The amount of time depends on several factors including the size and position of the baby at the start of the second stage. Your position will also affect how long it takes for the baby to be born.

Q WHY DOES THE SECOND STAGE TAKE THAT LONG?

A It takes time for the baby to rotate and fit through the pelvis. The baby moves down during the contraction and then slips back a bit after the contraction ends. This slow descent is useful because it gives the baby's head time to mold or change shape a bit, making it easier to fit through the pelvis. (See page 145 for more on newborn appearance.)

Q WHAT DOES IT MEAN WHEN THE BABY'S HEAD CROWNS?

A Crowning occurs when the baby's head no longer slips back between contractions. At this time the vaginal outlet is stretched to the maximum, which produces a stinging or burning sensation called the "rim of fire." This means the baby's head is about to be born.

Q WHY ARE YOU TOLD TO PANT OR BLOW OUT JUST BEFORE THE BABY'S HEAD IS BORN?

A It takes a lot of hard pushing to move the baby through the pelvis. However, when the baby's head is about to come through the vaginal outlet, it's better for it to gently slip through. If you lightly pant or blow out rather than push hard, you don't add to the force of the contractions. That makes it easier on your perineum (the area between your vagina and anus) and reduces the risk of tearing or extending an episiotomy. (See pages 109–110.) Your care provider will guide you, asking you to pant or give little pushes so the head eases out.

Q WHAT AM I SUPPOSED TO DO AFTER THE BABY'S HEAD IS OUT?

A You'll need to push a few more times to birth the rest of the baby's body. After the head is born, the baby's head turns toward the mother's leg. Then the shoulders and the rest of the body are born. The final step is for your care provider to clamp and cut the umbilical cord or ask your partner to cut it.

BIRTHING THE PLACENTA AND
IMMEDIATELY AFTER BIRTH

Q WHAT AM I SUPPOSED TO DO DURING THE THIRD STAGE?

A After the hard work of second stage, the third stage is considerably easier and shorter. It usually lasts less than 30 minutes and begins with a lull. First, your uterus rests a bit and then starts contracting. These contractions may feel like cramps, or you may not notice them at all. Their purpose is to detach the placenta from the wall of the uterus. Once that has happened, your care provider will ask you to start pushing again. It's much easier to push out the placenta (usually only a push or two).

Your care provider will catch the placenta in a pan and then examine it. If you and your partner are interested, you can ask your provider to show you the placenta, including the membranes and umbilical cord.

Q WHAT HAPPENS AFTER THE PLACENTA IS BORN?

A Your care provider and nurse will be attentive to your recovery. This includes monitoring your vital signs to make sure they return to normal. Your nurse will be checking your blood pressure, heart rate, and breathing. In addition, there are procedures to facilitate the postpartum healing process. These include making sure all the placenta has been expelled, repairing an episiotomy or tears, and making sure the uterus stays contracted.

Keeping your uterus contracted is important because when the uterus contracts, it seals off the blood vessels that supplied the placental site. This prevents excessive bleeding (postpartum hemorrhage). When your baby suckles at your breast, this will cause your uterus to contract. Between feedings, you can rub the top of your uterus to stimulate contractions. Ask your nurse to show you how to do this.

Your nurse may also put an ice pack against your perineum to help reduce swelling and to make you more comfortable.

Q WHAT ARE AFTERPAINS?

A These are the uterine contractions that occur after the baby and placenta are born. In the days after birth, they help the uterus return to its prepregnant size. In the beginning they feel like cramps. Some women find it helpful to use their breathing techniques during these contractions. You may also be offered a pain reliever such as ibuprofen or acetaminophen. After a few days you'll no longer feel these contractions. Women who are having their second or later baby have more painful cramping than first-time mothers.

Q HOW WILL I FEEL RIGHT AFTER THE BIRTH?

A If you didn't have an epidural or spinal analgesia, you may feel quite good because of the endorphins produced during labor. Endorphins are hormones that decrease pain and give you a sense of well-being. If you received an epidural or spinal analgesia, it may still be in effect. Some women feel exhausted right after birth, while others don't feel tired for several hours.

Over the next twelve hours or so, you'll probably become more aware of afterpains and a sore bottom. Some women have sore muscles from pushing or using certain labor positions. If you're uncomfortable, your care provider will order pain relievers that are safe for you to take.

Q WHAT IS LOCHIA?

A Lochia is the flow that's part of the recovery of your uterus. At the beginning this flow is bright red and contains some blood clots. Because this flow is like a heavy period, you'll need to wear a sanitary napkin. The birth facility will supply them during your stay. When you go home, you'll need a maxi-style pad. Do not use tampons. Over the next couple of weeks, the flow will decrease and become clearer. Breastfeeding speeds recovery because oxytocin, the hormone involved with the letdown of milk, also contracts the uterus. As a result, you produce less lochia than you would if you were formula feeding.

YOUR COPING STYLE

Q HOW CAN I TELL WHAT COPING TECHNIQUES WILL WORK FOR ME IN LABOR?

A Your coping style has evolved from your temperament and experiences. In labor you'll most likely respond in ways you normally use to cope with stress and physical discomfort. For example, if you usually prefer an undisturbed, quiet environment, your partner can help create and guard that space by reminding others not to interrupt you during a contraction. If you like to be distracted, you may find it helpful to focus on breathing, counting, or chanting. If you like to have someone take care of you, you may want your partner to give you physical support such as massaging your feet or slow dancing with you. If you like music or a warm bath, these may be appealing in labor. Although you may not prefer these techniques throughout your entire labor, they're the things to try first.

Q IS THERE SOMETHING I CAN TRY TO DISCOVER HOW I COPE WITH PAIN?

A Although holding ice doesn't really feel like a labor contraction, the ice-cube-minute is something you can try. The growing intensity of a sensation in one part of your body will allow you to test some coping measures. However, don't do this if you have a medical condition made worse by exposing your hands to cold.

When your partner is available and can keep track of the time, hold a handful of ice for 1 minute. Have your partner tell you when 20, 40, and 60 seconds have passed. You can do anything you want to cope with holding the ice, except pass it from hand to hand. Try to hold it for the full minute. If your hands have tough skin and holding the ice is not a challenge, put it against the inside of your wrist.

After the minute is up, put down the ice and discuss what you did. Also talk about what your partner noticed and what you wanted your partner to do. Then repeat the ice-cube-minute. After a few tries you'll have a good idea of what coping measures work for you.

Q I KNOW WHAT WORKED DURING THE ICE-CUBE-MINUTE, BUT HOW CAN I APPLY THAT TO LABOR?

A You can build on what you know about your coping style to better plan your labor environment.

- If you went deep inside yourself or went somewhere else in your mind, you may prefer to have your labor room be quiet and calm. This may include indirect lighting. Those with you shouldn't talk during contractions because you won't want to be pulled out of your concentration. Consider whether soft music may be helpful.
- If you moved your hand or arm, you may want to use labor positions that allow you to rock or sway your pelvis, such as slow dancing with your partner, rocking in a rocking chair, or gently bouncing on a birth ball.
- If you moved your body or walked around, it may be important for you not to be confined to a bed. That may mean choosing pain medication options that allow you to move.
- If you talked or vocalized, you're likely to do that in labor. Chanting or moaning will be ways of coping rather than signs of distress.
- If you kept your attention focused on the ice, you may want to do that with the contractions.
- If you were very deliberate and focused on something other than the ice, you'll probably find attention-focusing activities like distraction breathing, counting, or repeating a rhyme or verse helpful.

BREATHING

Q WHY DO SOME WOMEN LEARN BREATHING TECHNIQUES FOR LABOR?

A You can use breathing techniques to do two different things: to relax and to decrease discomfort or pain. Knowing how to decrease stress or discomfort through slow breathing is something you can use throughout your labor and throughout your lifetime. Many women find that concentrating on breathing is more helpful than concentrating on contractions. They also use breathing to help them cope with medical procedures.

Q HOW DO YOU DO DISTRACTION BREATHING?

A Although some women use slow, relaxation breathing as a focus throughout labor, most switch to lighter breathing when contractions get intense. Light, easy breathing is easier to pattern and change, making it more of a distraction. This kind of breathing doesn't have to be fast. It should be comfortably light and easy.

Distraction breathing works because you're concentrating on it. The fact that you're doing something is more important than what you're doing. Many women practice one style of breathing while they're pregnant and find themselves doing something else in labor. That's just fine. In labor, adapt your breathing however you need to.

There are different things you can do with your breathing. Experiment and decide which options you like best.

- The easiest distraction is to think the words *in* and *out* as you breathe in and out. This will help keep your breathing even. An alternative is to think the word *in* and say the word *out*.

- You can also count your breaths. It may be easier to softly count each exhalation until you reach four, then start over. You can choose any number you like. Most women find numbers six or under easiest to work with.

- Instead of counting, you can make a specific sound on each exhalation. The most common sounds are *hahh*, *ohh*, and *hee*. You can use the same sound on each exhalation or create a pattern of sounds such as three *hahhs* and a *hee*.

- Keep your breathing at a comfortable pace. Rather than speeding up your breathing, make the pattern of the exhaled sounds more complicated. This will prevent you from getting dizzy.

Q I LIKE THE IDEA OF CONCENTRATING ON SOMETHING, BUT I DON'T LIKE DOING BREATHING TECHNIQUES. WHAT ELSE CAN I DO?

A Instead of focusing on your breathing, focus on something else. Counting and rhythmic chanting are two common options. Some women concentrate on the clock or their watch, counting each second as it passes. Other women count things in the room like the corners of a picture frame or the pattern on the wallpaper. Chanting can be simple, such as saying "Out" with every exhalation or repeating a short prayer or the refrain of a song.

Q WHAT'S THE BEST TIME TO DO RELAXATION BREATHING?

A This will depend on your preference. Relaxation breathing during contractions, especially those in early labor, may be all you need to stay comfortable. When the contraction begins, start your relaxation breathing. Continue doing it until the contraction is over. Then breathe without focusing on your breath until the next contraction begins. Use this breathing for as long as it works.

As labor gets more intense, you may find it hard to relax between contractions. When your contractions are coming too close together to use other relaxation techniques, take a slow, deep breath at the end of a contraction, let it out, and use your relaxation breathing until the beginning of the next contraction. When that contraction begins, resume your distraction breathing or focusing technique. Labor is less exhausting when you can relax between contractions.

You can also do relaxation breathing whenever you begin to get tense. It may help you cope with events such as cervical checks and medical procedures.

TOUCH AND MASSAGE

Q I LIKE TO BE STROKED AND TOUCHED. WILL THAT BE COMFORTING IN LABOR?

A It may. Early in labor when you're trying to get relaxed and into a rhythm with your contractions, stroking may be quite helpful. Usually firm yet gentle strokes feel the best. You can decide where you want to be touched. Hand and foot massages can also be helpful. When the stroking is no longer soothing, your labor partner can use another form of support.

Q IS THERE ANY KIND OF TOUCH I CAN DO MYSELF?

A Try effleurage, or light stroking with the fingertips. You can stroke the skin of your belly or thighs directly, or you can cover the area with a sheet or piece of clothing. This kind of touch can be soothing and can take your mind off the contractions. You may also find that effleurage helps you relax between contractions.

Q I DON'T LIKE MASSAGES. WILL THAT BE A PROBLEM IN LABOR?

A No. Just tell your labor support people that you don't want to have your skin or hair stroked during labor. If you change your mind and want some kind of touch, you may find that a firm, steady holding of your shoulders or feet makes you feel more grounded or secure. Whenever a technique is no longer helpful, just tell the person.

PAIN MEDICATION

Q **WHAT SHOULD I THINK ABOUT WHEN CONSIDERING PAIN MEDICATION FOR LABOR?**

A It's helpful to identify your preferences regarding pain and pain medication while you're still pregnant. However, your final decision about pain medication is best made when you're in labor. That allows you to take into account the factors and events that may be affecting your experience. These include the size and position of your baby, how much progress was made before labor began, your current comfort level, how fast the labor is progressing, and your energy level. Here are some things to consider:

- What are your feelings about labor pain and pain medication? Some women want to avoid pain; others want to avoid pain medication.
- How does your partner feel? Sometimes a woman agrees to pain medication in order to make her partner feel more comfortable.
- How much support will you have during childbirth? Women who don't feel well supported often choose stronger pain medication.
- What kind of pain medication is most commonly used where you'll be giving birth? When you're in labor, it may feel easier to choose what's usually done. Additional labor support may help you feel more confident in your preference.
- What kind of pain medication does your care provider recommend or support? Care providers have their own preferences. Try to get your provider's support before you go into labor.

Q **WHAT KINDS OF PAIN MEDICATION ARE AVAILABLE FOR THE FIRST STAGE OF LABOR?**

A Because facilities vary in what they offer, ask your care provider or childbirth educator what's available. (See page 105 for a list of questions you can ask about pain medications.) One type of medication is a pain reliever that's given by injection, such as fentanyl or Nubain. It usually works for one to two hours and "takes the edge off" rather than providing complete relief.

Epidural analgesia is pain medication injected into the space around the spinal canal. An epidural combines a pain reliever with medication that numbs the nerves to the abdomen, lower back, and perineum. It may also affect the legs. An epidural often provides excellent pain control. A narrow tube remains in place throughout labor so additional medication can be given.

Spinal or intrathecal analgesia is a pain reliever injected into the spinal fluid. This provides very good pain relief with only a small amount of medication. It's usually given only once.

A paracervical block is medication to numb the cervix. It's injected into both sides of the cervix and blocks the pain of dilation. It doesn't affect other sources of pain.

Q WHAT ARE POSSIBLE PAIN-RELIEVING OPTIONS FOR SECOND STAGE?

A Epidurals and spinal analgesia are also effective for second stage. A pudendal block is medication that numbs the nerves of the vagina and perineum (the area between the vagina and anus). It's injected into both sides of the vagina. Nitrous oxide, or laughing gas, decreases pain awareness. The woman holds a mask and inhales the gas when she needs pain relief. A "local" or perineal anesthetic can be injected into the perineum to numb it before an episiotomy or repair.

Ten Questions to Ask about Pain Medications

1. What is it?
2. How does it work?
3. How will it make me feel?
4. How long does it last?
5. What has to be done before I can get it?
6. What are the side effects?
7. How will it affect my labor?
8. How will it affect my baby?
9. How soon can I get it?
10. When is the latest I can get it?

Q ALL OF MY FRIENDS HAD EPIDURALS. WHY DOESN'T EVERY WOMAN HAVE ONE?

A Because only anesthesiologists (and in some hospitals nurse anesthetists) place epidurals, they aren't always an option. Not all hospitals have these specialists immediately available twenty-four hours a day. In addition, not all women want an epidural because:

- Some do not want or need this level of pain control. They may prefer self-help comfort measures like breathing and relaxation instead.
- For some women, being able to move around is important. Even women with "light" epidurals usually stay in bed.
- An epidural may leave a woman feeling detached from her body and the birth process. Some women don't want that.
- Even though epidurals can help a woman feel in control of her response to labor, she has less control over the procedures she will experience. Epidurals require a considerable number of interventions including

intravenous (IV) fluids, electronic fetal monitoring, blood pressure monitoring, and perhaps cardiac monitoring and a urinary catheter. Epidurals also increase the likelihood that Pitocin will be needed and forceps or a vacuum extractor will be used.

- Although epidurals are safe, babies sometimes show subtle and temporary neurological effects from the medication. Epidurals also increase the risk of the baby being kept in the nursery because the mother had an elevated temperature. Although this is most likely a side effect of the epidural, care providers must make sure the baby doesn't have an infection. Some women don't want to take this risk.

Q **MY SISTER SAID SHE FELT QUITE ALONE AFTER SHE HAD HER EPIDURAL. WHAT CAN I DO TO PREVENT THAT?**

A Before a woman has an epidural for pain relief, she may need active support or coaching from her partner. Once the epidural is working, her lack of pain may be misinterpreted as her no longer needing support. Although she may not feel her contractions, she's still in labor and needs supportive attention.

When you and your partner talk about pain medication, also talk about your need for support. Discuss the fact that if you have an epidural, you would like your partner to stay close and give you attention. Talk about some of the things he or she can do to help you feel supported.

INDUCTION AND AUGMENTATION

Q HOW DOES LABOR INDUCTION WORK?

A Induction is starting labor before it starts on its own. The most common way to induce labor is to increase the amount of oxytocin in the woman's body. (Oxytocin is the hormone that makes the uterus contract.) Pitocin (the drug form of oxytocin) is given through an intravenous (IV) solution. The dosage is increased until the woman is having strong and frequent contractions. Sometimes another procedure, an amniotomy, is done, either alone or after the start of Pitocin. An amniotomy is also called artificial rupture of membranes (AROM). The breaking of the bag of waters usually moves the baby's head down, putting more pressure on the cervix. That can start contractions or make them stronger.

In order for an induction to be successful, the cervix needs to be ripe or soft. If the woman's cervix is not favorable for an induction, there are several things that can be done as the first step in an induction process. These involve stimulating the woman's body to make prostaglandins (hormones that soften or ripen the cervix). A care provider may use a finger to separate the membranes from the cervix (called stripping the membranes) or may apply a hormone preparation to the cervix. Sometimes these methods are enough to get labor started on their own.

If induction is needed, talk with your care provider about what methods will be best for you.

Q ARE THERE THINGS I CAN DO MYSELF TO HELP GET LABOR GOING?

A There are, but before you try them, talk with your care provider. Breast stimulation, especially the nipple area, can be a way to start labor. Brushing or rolling one (or both) nipples must be done gently because it may have to be done for several hours. Sexual foreplay and orgasm may cause contractions that stimulate labor. Semen contains prostaglandins that may help ripen the cervix. However, if your membranes have broken, you shouldn't have intercourse because of the risk of infection.

Acupressure and acupuncture work energy sites in the body and may stimulate contractions. Herbal preparations such as evening primrose oil may also cause contractions. These, however, need to be treated as medications because they enter the bloodstream and can affect the baby as well as the mother.

Q IF MY LABOR SLOWS DOWN, WHAT CAN BE DONE TO SPEED IT UP?

A Augmentation is the term for making contractions stronger. This is a way to speed up labor. Walking and upright positions can help stimulate a labor that's slowing. The stress response brought on by fear and pain can also slow labor. Addressing a woman's concerns and comfort needs may promote a more effective labor. In many cases a care provider uses Pitocin or an amniotomy. (See page 107.)

MONITORING

Q WHY IS IT IMPORTANT TO MONITOR A BABY'S HEART RATE IN LABOR?

A Care providers monitor the baby's well-being by the heart rate. Rates that are slower or faster than the normal 110–170 beats per minute can indicate the baby is having difficulty. How the baby's heart rate responds to contractions indicates how well the baby is handling the stress of labor.

Q WHO WILL MONITOR MY BABY'S HEART RATE?

A Most likely your nurse will do the monitoring. She'll report the results to your care provider. If you have a midwife, she may do the monitoring when she's with you.

Q HOW IS A BABY'S HEART RATE MONITORED IN LABOR?

A One method is by auscultation. A nurse or midwife monitors the baby's heart rate using a special stethoscope or a hand-held ultrasound device. This monitoring is done at regular intervals. It's effective yet allows the woman to move around and use comfort measures such as a shower. It does, however, require that a nurse or care provider be actively involved with every monitoring session. Some facilities aren't staffed for this.

Electronic fetal monitoring (EFM) is the other method. This kind of monitoring can be done by external or internal means. The external method monitors the baby's heart rate using ultrasound. A pressure-sensitive device tracks the mother's contractions. Two small monitors are positioned on the woman's abdomen and held in place by belts or stretchy material. The information is sent through wires to a machine that displays and records the results. Some hospitals eliminate the need for wires by using telemetry.

EFM provides continuous monitoring without a nurse always being present. Continuous monitoring is necessary during some medical procedures like induction. The disadvantages are that it restricts the mother's mobility and may limit her labor options.

Internal monitoring is used to get direct measurements. A small electrode attached to the baby's head monitors the baby's heart rate. This eliminates problems caused by the baby's or mother's movements. Internal monitoring requires that the bag of waters be broken and that the cervix be open a few centimeters. The mother's contractions may be monitored externally while this is taking place. Sometimes a pressure-sensitive probe is inserted into the uterus to monitor the contractions.

Eight Questions to Ask About a Procedure

1. What is it?
2. Why do I need it?
3. How does it work?
4. What will I feel?
5. How will it affect my baby?
6. How will it affect the rest of my care?
7. What are the other options?
8. How soon must I make a decision?

Q CAN I REQUEST A SPECIFIC METHOD OF MONITORING?

A Most birth facilities use electronic fetal monitoring (EFM) for 20–30 minutes when you first arrive. This is done to create a baseline reading that shows how the baby's heart is responding to contractions. Hospital policies differ on what's done after that. If you'd prefer not having EFM after the baseline is taken, talk with your care provider. That can be part of your birth plan. (See pages 118–120.) Continuous monitoring is necessary if you're given medications that can affect the baby, such as Pitocin and epidural pain medication.

EPISIOTOMY

Q WHY IS AN EPISIOTOMY NEEDED?

A An episiotomy is a cut to make the vaginal outlet larger. This is more often necessary when forceps or a vacuum extractor will be used. (See page 111.). It may also be done if there's concern that the vaginal outlet isn't large enough for the baby's head to fit through. Care providers vary in how frequently they do episiotomies. Some do them routinely, believing they're easier to repair than a tear. Others try to avoid them.

Most women don't feel the cut of the episiotomy. The pressure of the baby's head on the vaginal outlet temporarily numbs the area. The care provider injects a local anesthetic before doing the repair if the woman doesn't have pain medication already in effect. Absorbable stitches are used for the repair. That means they don't have to be removed.

Q HOW CAN I AVOID AN EPISIOTOMY?

A The first thing to do is talk with your care provider about your desire to avoid one. Discuss what preventive measures you can take while you're still pregnant. Some providers recommend massaging and gently stretching the perineum (the tissue between the vagina and anus). Your care provider may also do this just before the baby is born.

In addition, doing Super Kegel exercises during pregnancy makes the pelvic floor muscles more elastic. (See pages 64–65.) That allows them to stretch more easily during birth. Being aware of the muscles also helps you to consciously relax them when you push. This combination of relaxation and flexibility decreases the need for an episiotomy.

Your pushing position can also make a difference. A position like squatting helps keep pressure evenly distributed around the vaginal outlet. This helps the tissue stretch. Lying on your back with your legs held back pulls some of the tissue to the side, which makes it harder for the outlet to stretch evenly.

Q DOES EVERY WOMAN HAVE EITHER AN EPISIOTOMY OR A TEAR?

A Some women don't have either. Women having their second (or later) vaginal birth are less likely to have a tear or need an episiotomy. In addition, some tears are so small that they don't need stitching.

FORCEPS AND VACUUM EXTRACTOR

Q WHAT DO FORCEPS OR A VACUUM EXTRACTOR DO?

A Both can be used to guide a baby's head into a better position, enabling the baby to be born vaginally. Forceps look like two spoons placed on each side of the baby's head. During a contraction, the care provider uses the forceps to turn the baby's head or move it down. A vacuum extractor looks like a cap with a handle. It uses suction to keep the cap on the baby's head. The choice of method usually depends on the care provider's prefer- ence. Today more US care providers prefer a vacuum extractor.

An episiotomy and local (or regional) anesthesia may be needed when forceps or a vacuum extractor is used. Either technique may result in some vaginal bruising. Forceps may leave some bruising on the baby's face. A vacuum extractor raises a soft lump on the baby's head that looks like a large bruise. These disappear over time.

CESAREAN BIRTH

Q WHY IS A CESAREAN NEEDED?

A A cesarean is the birth of a baby by abdominal surgery. Cesareans are performed for a number of reasons, the most common being the fail- ure of labor to progress. That may mean the cervix stops dilating or there's too little labor progress even after efforts have been made to strengthen con- tractions. At other times the membranes break prematurely and the woman's body doesn't go into labor. Another reason for lack of progress is that the baby's head stays high in the pelvis. This is known as cephalo-pelvic dis- proportion (CPD). Sometimes this happens because of the baby's position. Other times the size of the baby's head or the shape of the mother's pelvis prevents the baby from descending.

A second cause for cesarean birth is fetal distress. This means the baby's heart rate indicates the baby is having trouble handling labor. Most providers advise a cesarean if the heart rate doesn't improve with a change in the mother's position or with other simple measures.

A third cause is the woman's last baby was born by cesarean and the woman and her care provider have decided to schedule a repeat cesarean.

There are also less common causes. The presentation of the baby, such as a feet-first breech, may indicate the need for a cesarean. Twins are often born by cesarean because one or both of them may be breech or in a poor position for vaginal birth. If the mother has a medical condition, such as heart trouble, a cesarean may be done for the mother's health. Or it may be done to protect the baby's health. This can happen when the mother has an infection, such as a herpes outbreak, or if there's a problem with the placenta.

Often the reason for a first cesarean doesn't repeat itself in the next pregnancy. Then, the woman and her care provider may choose a vaginal birth after cesarean (VBAC). (See page 125.)

Q WOULDN'T IT BE EASIER TO SKIP LABOR AND JUST HAVE A CESAREAN?

A A cesarean is usually a safe birth option. The baby's or mother's health may require it. However, a cesarean isn't the best option in all circumstances. Although it may sound appealing to avoid labor and go right to the baby's birth, there are drawbacks.

A woman who has had a cesarean not only has to adapt to postpartum body changes, she has to recover from major abdominal surgery. This affects her mobility and ability to care for her baby after birth. Recovery is slower and more painful than with a vaginal birth. In addition, some women get an infection or other problem that further slows their recovery. Having several cesareans may increase the risk of a problem with the placenta in a future pregnancy.

An additional consideration is that labor plays a role in a newborn's transition to breathing. The normal stress of the contractions stimulates hormones in the baby that help clear fluid from the lungs after birth. Pressure on the baby's chest during vaginal birth also helps get rid of fluid. As a result, babies born vaginally are less likely to have breathing problems right after birth.

In terms of total ease, a vaginal birth is easier. If your concerns go beyond ease, share them with your care provider. There may be birth options that make labor seem more doable for you.

Q HOW CAN I AVOID A CESAREAN BIRTH?

A cesarean birth may be necessary in certain circumstances. For example, the position of the placenta may make vaginal birth impossible. However, there are things you can do to increase the likelihood of a vaginal birth:

• Maintain a healthy lifestyle. Eliminate the possibility that complications from tobacco or drug use, for example, will require your baby to be born before labor starts.

• Keep all your prenatal appointments. This makes it easier to treat a problem if one develops. For example, treating an infection may prevent the premature breaking of the bag of waters.

• Avoid having labor induced for a nonmedical reason. Wait until your body is ready to go into labor.

• Unless your care provider tells you not to, stay home until labor is well established. Going to the hospital early in labor may mean spending most of your time in bed. This may result in a slow labor. Interventions used to speed up your labor may increase the risk of a cesarean.

• Consider pain-relief alternatives that don't require you to remain in bed. When you're able to move around, you can use movement to help your baby get into a better position for birth.

• If you've had an epidural, let it wear off enough to feel your body's messages to push. If that isn't possible, some care providers advise not pushing until the baby's head can be seen at the vaginal outlet. These techniques reduce the need for a cesarean as well as forceps or a vacuum extractor. (See page 111.)

CHILDBIRTH CLASSES

Q ARE CHILDBIRTH CLASSES WORTHWHILE?

A Yes, they are. However, childbirth classes vary in their philosophies, teaching methods, and formats. It's important to choose a class that meets your needs.

Q WHAT SHOULD I CONSIDER WHEN LOOKING FOR A CHILDBIRTH CLASS?

A Most childbirth classes cover basic information about birth and birth-related procedures. However, they vary in how the information is presented and how much time is spent on comfort measures. Some classes also cover breastfeeding and parenting a newborn.

Classes offered by a hospital, birth center, or care provider will provide information regarding the policies and procedures of that facility or practice. Independent educators or childbirth education groups may promote a specific philosophy like the Bradley method or Lamaze normal birth. Others may be more like the International Childbirth Education Association (ICEA) and promote family-centered birth. You may also be able to find specialty classes. These include birth taught in the context of a religion and classes for a specific group like teens, same-sex couples, and families who have had a prior birth experience.

Class sizes and schedules also vary. When the class has no more than ten couples, it's easier to get to know each other and ask questions. A series taught over five or six weeks gives you time to practice the skills and develop relationships. A weekend class concentrates the information into a single weekend, which may benefit couples who have scheduling conflicts. Private education can tailor a class to your specific needs. (See page 115 for questions to ask about the educator and class.)

Q HOW CAN I FIND CLASSES IN MY AREA?

A You can locate classes by:
- Talking to your care provider;
- Contacting your hospital or birth center or checking their website;
- Asking friends and colleagues;

- Looking online for a list of instructors certified by national childbirth organizations. For example, you can visit www.icea.org, www.lamaze.org, and www.bradleybirth.com.
- Checking maternity and baby supply stores for a list of community birth resources.

Questions to Ask a Childbirth Educator or Education Coordinator

- What is your philosophy of childbirth?
- What topics do you cover?
- How are classes organized?
- How much time is spent on lecture, discussion, and practice?
- What's the class schedule and location?
- How many participants are likely to be in the class?
- What's the maximum number?
- What's the cost?
- Are there scholarships?
- Do you offer other kinds of childbirth or parenting classes?
- If I have a special circumstance, how will this be accommodated?
- Are you (or the educator) a certified childbirth educator? If so, by what organization?
- What other professional qualifications do you (or the instructor) have, such as nurse, lactation consultant, or early childhood development specialist?

BIRTH DOULAS

Q WHAT IS A DOULA?

A A doula is a professional who provides support to a laboring woman and her partner. Doulas vary in the specific services they provide, but they all provide physical, emotional, and informational support. They do not provide medical or nursing care. Most doulas are private and hired by the pregnant woman. A few hospitals have doulas on staff.

The advantage of a private doula is that you meet with her one or more times during your pregnancy to talk about childbirth and the role you'd like her to play. Then, when labor begins, you contact her. Some doulas come to your home; others meet you at the hospital or birth center. The cost of a private doula varies by location and the services provided. Nationally, fees range from $200–$850. Some doulas are able to offer a sliding fee scale or reduced rate for those who need it. Not many insurance plans cover doula services. It's important to interview potential doulas as early as possible in the pregnancy because each doula limits the number of clients she accepts. (See page 117 for interview questions.)

Hospital-based doulas usually meet you for the first time when you're admitted to the hospital. Although the doula will not have met you before-hand to do birth planning, she can provide effective support based on your preferences. Because she's part of the staff, she'll be familiar with hospital procedures. The cost varies by the type of program the hospital establishes. Contact the facility you'll be using to find out if they have a doula service and what it entails.

Q WHAT ARE THE ADVANTAGES OF HAVING A DOULA?

A Having a doula can increase your sense of control, which can increase your satisfaction with your birth experience. Although you can't control the course of your labor, you can affect how the decisions are made. This may enable you to have the best birth experience possible. A doula's positive influence may also carry over into the postpartum period. In some studies, women who had been supported by a doula had less postpartum depression, a more positive view of their babies, and breastfed their babies longer. A vast majority of women who are supported by a doula say they would have a doula at their next birth. A doula provides support and increases your satisfaction by:

- Giving you continuous attention and support;
- Informing you about the labor and birth process;
- Working with you to increase your emotional and physical comfort;
- Suggesting comfort measures or coping techniques;
- Helping your partner help you;
- Helping you develop questions to ask your nurse or care provider so you can better understand a choice or decision you have to make;
- Acting as your advocate.

For more information on doulas, visit the Doulas of North America (DONA) website at www.dona.org. The International Childbirth Education Association (ICEA) also certifies doulas. Visit www.icea.org.

Q WHY WOULD I WANT A DOULA WHEN MY PARTNER WILL BE WITH ME?

A Your partner brings the power of love and a shared history that provide a unique and important kind of support. However, most partners don't know a lot about the birth process and aren't skilled at providing physical support. That can leave them feeling helpless and isolated when they're the sole support person. Partners also have their own concerns about childbirth, being in a hospital, and seeing their loved one in labor. Partners find doulas helpful because they provide information, make suggestions about comfort techniques, and provide support for the partner's needs such as enabling him or her to take a break.

Q WON'T MY NURSE PROVIDE THE SUPPORT I NEED WHEN I'M IN THE HOSPITAL?

A Only a few hospitals have sufficient staff to provide a laboring woman with one-to-one nursing care throughout labor. Even if this is available, the nurse's primary responsibility is your healthcare. Many of her duties require her to focus on procedures or take her out of the room. As a result, she won't be able to provide continuous emotional and physical support. In addition, nurses work by shift, so you may have more than one nurse during your labor. A doula focuses solely on providing you with support and stays with you throughout your labor and birth.

Q I'D LIKE TO HAVE A DOULA BUT CAN'T FIND ONE IN MY AREA.

A There are two different approaches you can take. One is to find a female friend or relative who could be a support person. Although this

Questions to Ask a Doula

- What services do you provide?
- What is your approach to providing support?
- How long have you been a doula?
- How many births have you attended?
- How did you get your training?
- Are you certified? Through what organization?
- How many births do you schedule in a month?
- Who will be the backup if you can't be at my birth? Will I get to meet her?
- Have you provided support in the hospital or birth center I'm using?
- Have you worked with my care provider or care provider's practice?
- What is your fee? How does it get paid?
- How many times will we meet during my pregnancy?
- What will happen in those visits?
- Will you come to my home in early labor?
- What comfort supplies do you bring (birth ball, music, aromatherapy, massage oil)?
- Will you take photographs? Do you bring your own camera?
- How long will you stay after the birth?
- Do you make a postpartum visit? When will that be? What will you do?
- Are you a certified lactation consultant?
- If there are special circumstances, have you ever provided support in a similar circumstance?

person won't be an expert, her familiar presence will go a long way toward making you and your partner feel more comfortable. When looking at possible candidates, consider the following:

- Are both you and your partner comfortable with the person? Tension among people in the room can make coping with labor harder.
- What childbirth experiences does the person have? It's beneficial if the person is familiar with the childbirth process, although it isn't essential for the person to have given birth.
- Does the person have a positive view of childbirth? Someone who has had a negative experience could cloud your experience with her own fears or memories.
- Will the person be available at any time?

The other approach is to ask someone who has a professional knowledge of birth but hasn't been trained as a doula.

- If you're taking prenatal classes, ask your instructor if she knows of someone who would be willing to provide labor support.
- Call the childbirth education coordinator at the hospital you're using, or contact a local childbirth education group. Many childbirth educators need to attend births as part of their certification or recertification.
- Contact the labor and birth area of your hospital or birth center. Sometimes the staff knows of nurses or midwives who would be available.
- Contact a local nursing or midwifery school. These students are often looking for such an opportunity.

BIRTH PLAN

Q **WHY MAKE A BIRTH PLAN WHEN I DON'T KNOW WHAT WILL HAPPEN IN LABOR?**

A A birth plan is not a set of rules or orders for labor. It's an explanation of your concerns, preferences, and priorities. Identifying what's most important to you helps both you and your care providers keep those things in focus. A birth plan doesn't dictate or interfere with your care. Instead, it helps others better understand what you want and need.

Q **HOW DO YOU MAKE A BIRTH PLAN?**

A The first step is to discuss your priorities with your partner. It may be best to begin by defining in broad terms how you view childbirth.

Think about the role you'd like to play in the decision making, how you view possible medical procedures, and how you see yourself coping with pain.

From there you can more easily describe your laboring preferences, including comfort measures and pushing techniques. You don't need to create a long list of preferences, but do mention anything that's particularly important. Also, think about what you'd like to be able to do right after your baby is born. This could include how you'd like to interact with your baby and how the staff can help with that. Because about one in six labors ends in a first-time cesarean, you and your partner should consider what would be most important if you had one.

You may want to review pages 90–99 on labor, pages 111–113 on cesarean birth, and pages 145–147 on baby's first hour after birth. You can also read more about birth options in *Pregnancy, Childbirth, and the Newborn* (by Simkin, Whalley, and Keppler) or visit a childbirth or healthcare website such as www.healthatoz.com or www.childbirth.org. You can also ask your childbirth educator or doula what's likely to be available at your birth facility.

How to Use Your Birth Plan Effectively in Labor

- Limit your plan to no more than one page.
- Use large type, bullets, and phrases so it can be read easily and quickly.
- Bring several copies to the hospital or birth center.
- Ask your nurse to put one copy in your chart.
- To make sure everyone sees your plan, post another copy in your room. A good place is at the sink or hand-washing area.
- Talk with your nurse about your birth plan.
- When you have to make a decision, ask how each option will affect your preferences.
- If something causes a change in plans, try to be flexible. Use your plan to stay focused on what's most important.

Then, write a draft of your birth plan. Use terms like "I (or we) prefer," "as much as possible," and "as a last resort" rather than "I want" or "we don't want." You'll sound less demanding, which will make it easier for others to honor your preferences. In addition, there's an understanding that requests are always on condition that the health of the mother and baby permit such an action. If you have concerns about birth or need reassurance because of a past event, include this in your birth plan to help your nurse and care provider better address that need.

After you share your birth plan with your doctor or midwife, create a final draft and ask that it be placed in your medical record.

Q HOW DO I PRESENT MY BIRTH PLAN TO MY CARE PROVIDER?

A Some providers are in favor of birth plans; others are not. Let your care provider know ahead of time that you'd like to discuss your birth preferences. Then use your plan as a way to begin the dialogue. If possible, have your partner come to that visit. The best strategy is to focus on what's most important to you. It may take more than one visit to talk through your priorities and concerns. Also, you may need to be flexible about some of your preferences and adapt your plan accordingly. The goal is for both you and your provider to feel comfortable with your birth plan.

If something you want is not commonly done, ask your provider what can be done to increase the likelihood of the request being honored. Consider asking your provider to write in your chart that he or she supports that preference. If you see several providers in a group practice, make sure to talk to each of them about your plan.

THE HOSPITAL TOUR

Q SINCE I'VE ALREADY TALKED WITH MY CARE PROVIDER ABOUT MY BIRTH PLAN, IS THERE ANY REASON TO TAKE A HOSPITAL TOUR?

A The tour will provide helpful information that you may not receive from other sources. Tours usually answer basic questions like:
• Where should I park?
• What door should I use?
• Do I have to stop at an admitting station?
• Is there a telephone in the room?
• Is there a refrigerator and a microwave I can use?
• Is there a shower or tub I can use?
• Is flash photography allowed in the labor or birthing rooms?

In addition, a tour lets you visit the labor-and-birth area so it will be familiar to you and your partner when you return in labor. Also, seeing a labor or birthing room may help you determine what you'll need to bring. Being together in the place where your baby will be born may provide an opportunity for you and your partner to talk and dream about your baby's birth.

Check with your facility to find out how tours are scheduled. You may need to register for a tour even if there isn't a fee.

PACKING LISTS

Q WHAT SHOULD I TAKE TO THE HOSPITAL?

A If you don't want to actually pack your bag, it's helpful to create a packing list early in your last month of pregnancy. That way if labor starts unexpectedly, you or someone else will know what to bring. However, if you leave without your bag, you'll still be able to manage labor with what the facility provides. Some women go through childbirth and never open their labor bag.

The following is a list of things to consider taking to the hospital or birth center. Take only the things that appeal to you or that apply to your situation.

For Labor:
- Insurance information, even if you've preregistered
- A large shirt or long top
- Socks to keep your feet warm
- Slippers
- Glasses
- If you wear contacts, contact case and solution
- Toiletries, especially toothbrush and toothpaste, comb or brush, and scrunchies to hold back your hair
- Lip balm
- Your pillow in a colorful pillowcase (Three or four are even better.)
- Cornstarch, unscented lotion, or massage oil
- CDs or cassette tapes and a CD/cassette player, if one isn't provided
- A photograph or small object to focus on
- Rice sock (tube sock filled with rice and sewn closed, which can be heated in the microwave)
- Small, frozen blue-ice pack
- Tennis balls to use when applying pressure to your back

For Your Partner:
- Comfortable shoes
- Swimsuit, if labor area has a shower, Jacuzzi, or spa tub
- Change of clothes
- Toiletries
- Food, including protein snacks and water or juice
- Change for vending machine

- Telephone numbers and calling card (Cell phones are often not allowed or don't work in a hospital.)
- Camera loaded with high-speed film or a full memory card and spare camera batteries

For Your Postpartum Stay:
- Nursing nightgown or pajamas
- Robe
- One or two nursing bras
- Maternity underwear
- Toiletries
- Comfortable outfit to wear home (Your abdomen is likely to be about the size it was when you were five months pregnant.)

For the Baby:
- Diapers
- Undershirt or onesie
- One-piece outfit
- Receiving blanket
- Hat
- Sweater or outside blanket, if weather is cool
- Car seat properly installed (You can't take a baby home in a car if you don't have a car seat.)

PRETERM LABOR

Q WHAT IS PRETERM LABOR?

A It's labor that starts between the 20th and 37th week of pregnancy, before the baby is at "term." The problem is that a baby born prematurely may need considerable help to survive. How much help depends on how premature the baby is. (See below for warning signs of preterm labor.)

Q HOW CAN I PREVENT PRETERM LABOR?

A It's important to keep all your prenatal appointments. That way your care provider can monitor your health and treat any problems as soon as they appear. Infections in the vagina or mouth have been identified as potential causes of preterm labor. Dehydration can also trigger contractions. Make sure you're getting at least eight cups of fluid each day, and even more if you live in a dry climate or are physically active. For more information on preterm labor, visit the March of Dimes website at www.marchofdimes.com/prematurity.

Q WHAT SHOULD I DO IF I THINK I'M HAVING PRETERM LABOR?

A If you're having signs that you may be in preterm labor, call your care provider's office. You may be told to drink 16 ounces of water and lie down on your left side. Then, monitor your contractions over the next hour or so. Sometimes resting and giving your body fluids will stop the contractions. If not, follow your care provider's instructions. These early contractions can often be stopped by medication. However, once labor gets established, contractions can usually only be delayed rather than stopped.

Warning Signs of Preterm Labor

- Contractions that are 10 minutes apart or less
- Regular tightening or pain in the lower abdomen or back
- Pressure in the pelvis or vagina
- Bleeding from the vagina
- Fluid leaking from the vagina
- A sense that things aren't right

MOTHER'S HEALTH

**Q I HAVE GENITAL HERPES.
WILL MY BABY HAVE TO BE BORN BY CESAREAN?**

A Most care providers recommend a cesarean if a woman is having an outbreak when she goes into labor. This prevents the baby from coming in contact with a lesion. Your provider may take a culture or look for signs that an outbreak may occur near your due date or when labor begins. If the virus isn't active, a vaginal birth is often an option. Ask your care provider what steps will be taken as your due date nears.

**Q I JUST TESTED POSITIVE FOR GROUP B STREP. I DIDN'T EVEN
KNOW I HAD IT. HOW WILL THAT AFFECT MY LABOR?**

A Some women are carriers of Group B streptococcus (GBS). That means the bacteria can be found in the genital area. Although a mother may not have any symptoms, GBS may possibly cause a life-threatening infection in her newborn. As a precaution, you'll probably be given an intravenous (IV) antibiotic when you're in labor. Your baby may also be given an antibiotic after birth. There is some variation in how care providers treat GBS, so make sure to talk with your provider.

PERSONAL CONCERNS

**Q I HAVE SOME EVENTS IN MY PAST THAT I WORRY MAY
AFFECT MY BIRTH. WHAT SHOULD I DO?**

A Share your concerns with your doctor or midwife. Be as frank as you can about your past. Your care provider may be able to allay some of your concerns. Consider asking for a referral to a counselor who has experience working with birth-related issues.

If your partner doesn't already know about your concerns, try to share them. Even if you can't talk about the past, talk about your concerns about birth. Then the two of you can make plans to have as much support on hand as possible. In addition, create a birth plan that describes how the nursing staff can help you. For example, you might ask for advance notice of any procedure so you have enough time to prepare for it.

Consider hiring a doula. (See pages 115–118.) If you're uncomfortable sharing your past, share only your concerns about birth. An experienced doula can provide effective labor support without knowing the basis for the concern.

VBAC

Q WHAT DOES *VBAC* MEAN?

A VBAC stands for vaginal birth after cesarean. Women who have had a baby by cesarean can often deliver their next baby vaginally. Some care providers promote VBACs; others do not. Whether a woman labors for a vaginal birth with her next baby depends on several factors including her feelings about another cesarean birth, where the scar is on her uterus, what caused the first cesarean, and the capabilities of her birth facility.

If you had a cesarean and are considering a VBAC, it will be helpful to write a birth plan and have good labor support as well as the support of your care provider. Consider reading *The VBAC Companion* by Diana Korte or visiting www.vbac.com. Your hospital or care provider may also offer a VBAC class.

UNDERSTANDING POST PARTUM

Q HOW LONG WILL IT TAKE FOR THINGS TO GET BACK TO NORMAL AFTER I GIVE BIRTH?

A They won't get *back* to normal. You'll achieve a new normal. The amount of time this takes depends on what you're considering. Your uterus will involute (return to nearly its prepregnant size) in about six weeks. However, most other aspects of post partum take considerably longer. By six months many mothers feel like they've mastered the caregiving tasks and have developed a strong relationship with their baby. They're now ready to look beyond the baby. At one year most mothers feel that they can deal with all the tasks they have to do in a day. This longer timeline for post partum reflects the fact that it's complex and involves more than the involution of the uterus.

Q WHY DOES POST PARTUM TAKE SO LONG?

A It takes a long time because there are a lot of things to accomplish. In addition to healing physically, you need to master caregiving tasks, adapt emotionally to being a mother, form a secure relationship with your baby, and redefine your other relationships, especially the one with your partner. All of these tasks have to be done at the same time, and each interacts with the others. If a problem develops, say in physical recovery, it slows the progress in all the other areas. Adding to the challenge is the fact that your baby keeps changing. This affects both your relationship with your baby and your mastery of caregiving tasks. For more information on the work of post partum, see *Postpartum: The Making of a Family* by Linda Todd, available through www.icea.org.

Q WHAT MAKES THE FIRST MONTH OF POST PARTUM HARD?

A For most new parents, the first month is a quest for sleep. Because a baby usually sleeps only a few hours at a time, you don't get any long stretches of sleep. It's very difficult to feel rested when your sleep is interrupted several times a night. In addition, most women enter post partum with a sleep deficit because of the discomforts of late pregnancy. Partners are overtired because they often need to keep their regular work schedule and have no opportunity to take even a short nap during the day. Being overtired makes it hard to cope with stress, and new parenting is stressful.

DEVELOPING A SUPPORT NETWORK

Q WHAT CAN MAKE THE FIRST MONTH OF POST PARTUM EASIER?

A Two things: limiting the demands on your time and energy, and having a support network. It's important that you take good care of yourself so that you can recover from childbirth. If you had a difficult vaginal birth or cesarean, that will increase your physical recovery time. In addition to healing, you'll need time to establish breastfeeding or formula feeding and build your relationship with your baby. The more you can reduce household tasks and limit outside responsibilities, the better. This will give you time and energy to devote to healing and feeling competent as a mother.

The other thing you'll need is support—both practical and emotional. As part of adjusting to motherhood, you'll want to talk about your baby's birth. That means having someone other than your partner to hear your birth story. Caring for a new baby is not only time consuming, it requires new skills. If this is your first baby, you'll likely have many questions. It's extremely helpful to have resources you can call on. In addition, it's reassuring to have someone affirm that you're being a good parent. Spend time before your baby is born identifying your support network. (See page 131.) Write down their names and telephone numbers, and post this list beside the phone or on the refrigerator so it's available when you need it.

Q WHAT DOES A MOTHERS' GROUP DO?

A A mothers' group (or a new moms' group) provides peer support. Because the group members are all facing the challenge of being a mother, they can give each other advice and support. The group also provides an opportunity to build friendships. As a result, the group can be tremendously helpful in easing a new mother's feelings of being overwhelmed and isolated.

Most groups begin with an experienced leader who facilitates the group's development. The early meetings usually have a specific topic plus time to talk about other things. In some groups the leader leaves after six to eight meetings. Then the group carries on by itself, although it may get smaller over time. Some of these groups continue to meet for years. In more formal programs, mothers graduate to different groups as their babies grow older. Many of these programs support mothers throughout their baby's first year.

It's best to sign up for a group before your baby is born. That way you'll have done the work of finding a group before you need one. It's very hard in the weeks after the birth to focus on the task of finding something new. You may be able to find a group through:

- Your childbirth educator;
- Your birth facility;
- Your care provider;
- Your religious group;
- Your community newspaper;
- Your local library;
- A pregnancy and parenting resource center;
- Local parenting publications;
- Childcare cooperatives.

Support groups are also available online. Conduct an Internet search using the words "mothers' groups." These sites don't offer the same opportunities for building personal relationships and don't get you out of the house. In addition, it may be hard to determine the source of the information and whether it's accurate. However, these sites do cover the issues new mothers face and they give people an opportunity to share.

Q I CAN'T FIND A MOMS' GROUP NEAR ME AND I DON'T KNOW OTHER NEW MOMS. WHAT CAN I DO?

A You may be able to develop a support network by rekindling old friendships with women who are now mothers. In addition, start introducing yourself to expectant or new mothers at your place of worship, workplace, or prenatal class. Go for a walk or to a nearby children's park and introduce yourself to a mother with an infant. Most mothers with infants are starved for adult conversation. The two of you will probably start talking about your babies. At the end of the conversation, you can decide whether you want to share phone numbers or plan to meet again.

You can also start your own group. That, however, requires time and energy. Your baby will probably be around six months old before you feel ready to take on such a task.

Q I'M A SINGLE MOTHER. WHAT DIFFERENCE WILL THAT MAKE DURING POST PARTUM?

A The biggest difference is you'll be responsible for everything. You'll need to draw on your support network so you don't become exhausted and overwhelmed. Consider asking family or friends to help you in the early weeks. Many people are delighted to help after the birth of a baby, so do try to ask for the help you need. In addition:

- Try to get out of the house each day. Take a walk with your baby. You'll benefit from the physical activity and from not feeling confined.
- Get into a group with other mothers, such as a new moms' group, an exercise or yoga class, or a single mothers' support group.

Identifying Your Support Network

Who will listen to your birth story? This person needs to be a good listener who will not jump in with her own story before you've told yours. Possibilities include:

- A female friend or relative;
- Your childbirth educator;
- Your doula;
- Your midwife.

Who will give you emotional support and reassure you that you're being a good parent? This person needs parenting experience or experience working with parents. Possibilities include:

- Your mother or mother-in-law, if she can identify with today's parenting styles and issues;
- A friend or relative;
- Your postpartum doula;
- Your baby's healthcare provider.

Who will give you expert advice about your baby's health? Possibilities include:

- Your baby's healthcare provider;
- Your pediatric provider's call-in service;
- An advice line provided by a children's hospital.

Who will give you expert advice on breastfeeding? Possibilities include:

- A lactation consultant;
- A La Leche League leader.

Who will give you help with household tasks? Possibilities include:

- Family or friends;
- Neighbors;
- Members of your religious group;
- Your postpartum doula;
- Housecleaning and shopping services.

- Ask for or give yourself gifts of a massage, manicure, or pedicure. Even a ten-minute chair massage feels great.
- Have a friend or two help with the housework. You can enjoy each other and the baby while the work gets done. In addition, consider slipping off for a long shower or bath. Then order takeout and enjoy a meal together.
- If you can afford it, purchase services. Having someone else do the laundry or clean your home may make your life feel less overwhelming. Many postpartum doulas will come at night. Having another person do some of the nighttime or early morning duties can give you more time to sleep.

PLANNING FOR THE BASICS

Q MY PARTNER AND I ARE TRYING TO DECIDE IF WE SHOULD HAVE ONE OF OUR MOTHERS COME AND HELP RIGHT AFTER THE BABY IS BORN.

A As you discuss your options, focus on who will make the early weeks the most comfortable for you. Look for someone who will take care of household tasks so you can concentrate on the baby. Family dynamics can be complicated, however. Here are some things to consider:

- Will your mother or mother-in-law be helpful or will she generate needs you have to meet?
- What do you want her to do?
- What has she said she wants to do?
- Will she compete with you for the baby?
- How well do you communicate with her?
- Is there normally tension when she visits?
- How have you resolved tense situations in the past?
- Does her coming complicate other family relationships?
- If she doesn't come, what are your alternatives?

You won't have the energy to care for her needs, too. If you think you may clash over parenting issues, have her come when you feel more secure in your parenting. For example, ask her to come at the end of the first month rather than the beginning. By then you'll feel less vulnerable but will still welcome the extra pair of hands.

Q MY PARTNER AND I DON'T HAVE ANYONE TO COME AND HELP US AFTER THE BABY IS BORN. WHAT KINDS OF PLANS SHOULD WE MAKE?

A Both of you can write down the things you'll need in order to function during the first month after your baby is born. Start with food and sleep. Then, after you've made your lists, compare them. Agree on how you'll attempt to accomplish the most important things. Be realistic. Your partner can't take over running the household if he or she has never done much of the work. If your partner has to return to work, there will be little time to do housework. First-time mothers can't be expected to do much more than take care of the baby in the first month. Mothers who have other children will need to focus on them as well as the baby.

You'll need to be creative. Consider ways to cut corners and let housework slide. For example, buy food that only needs reheating, or use paper products so you have fewer dishes. Consider hiring a postpartum doula, a housecleaning service, or a diaper service. Agree to put your energies toward what's most important to both of you. Most families with newborns have a pile of laundry on the couch and dirty dishes in the sink. If you had a neat home before the baby, you eventually will again.

As you start to get your energy back, agree on what should have priority. Consider taking turns: One person cares for the baby while the other works on something that's become irritating because it's no longer getting done, like vacuuming.

Q I KNOW FRIENDS WILL BE BRINGING OVER SOME DINNERS, BUT WHAT WILL I EAT DURING THE DAY? MY SISTER SAID SHE COULD NEVER FIND TIME TO EAT AND TAKE CARE OF THE BABY.

A If you're home alone with the baby during the day, you'll need a supply of food that's portable and ready to eat. Consider having your partner or a friend shop for some of the following:
- Yogurt
- Prepared vegetables and fruits (Supermarkets may sell these at a salad bar or in the produce section.)
- Protein bars
- Whole-grain cereals (You can eat these right out of the box as well as with milk.)
- Dried fruits and trail mix
- Nuts (walnuts, almonds, or cashews) and nut butters
- Whole-wheat pita bread and hummus
- Bran-based muffins that contain grated carrot and dried fruit
- Whole-grain crackers and cheese
- Fruit that's easy to eat, such as grapes or apples
- 100 percent fruit or vegetable juice
- Premade yogurt smoothies

In addition, fill a sports bottle with ice and water and put it near the chair you usually use when feeding your baby. That way you'll have something to drink close at hand.

PHYSICAL RECOVERY

Q HOW LONG WILL MY BOTTOM BE SORE?

A If you have stitches, they'll dissolve in 1–2 weeks. It will probably take 4–6 weeks for the tissues to heal. It's common to have some discomfort for up to 4–6 months. Many women, however, feel considerably less tender when they sit and walk 7–10 days after giving birth.

Tips for Getting Sleep

- Make getting sleep a priority. Try to rest whenever your baby is sleeping.
- Babies usually have one sleep period that's longer than the others. Try to sleep then so you can get as much sleep as possible at one time. Many babies develop a somewhat predictable sleep pattern that will guide you.
- Stay dressed for rest until you've gotten the sleep you need for the day. Staying in your sleepwear sends a reminder to yourself and others that you need to rest. If you don't want to remain in your sleepwear, choose clothing that's comfortable to sleep in.
- Make your bedroom a place for sleep. Don't turn on the TV. Turn the phone ringer off. Keep the room darkened when you're trying to sleep during the day. If your baby's sounds and movements keep you awake, consider putting the crib or bassinette in another room.
- If you're breastfeeding:
  * Take advantage of the calming effects of breastfeeding and go back to sleep as soon as the feeding is over. Ask your partner or support person to change the baby and settle her.
  * Consider keeping the bassinette next to your bed so you can slip your baby into the bassinette at the end of the feeding.
  * If someone is staying with you, ask that person to take the last night shift or first morning shift. Having someone else take care of the baby after a feeding means you can stay in bed.
- If you're formula feeding:
  * Alternate nights with your partner regarding who will feed and take care of the baby. That way one of you can get more sleep.
  * Consider asking someone else to feed the baby so you can sleep through that feeding.

Hemorrhoids usually shrink in 2–4 weeks. Avoiding constipation will promote healing. If you're still bothered by them at the time of your postpartum visit, you and your provider can talk about treatment options. The following techniques promote comfort and healing for sore tissues and hemorrhoids:

- Sit with your feet up, or lie down as often as possible. This decreases swelling.
- Use cold to decrease swelling and increase comfort. This includes ice packs, sanitary pads soaked in witch hazel and chilled in the freezer, Tucks (witch hazel pads) chilled in the refrigerator, and sitz baths (sitting in a shallow bath) in cold water.
- Use warmth to increase blood flow and speed healing. This includes warm packs and sitz baths in comfortably warm water.
- Keep the area clean. After urinating, pour water over the area. This is easy to do if you use a squeeze bottle. Always wipe from front to back.
- Start doing Kegel exercises (tightening then relaxing your pelvic floor muscles). When you feel you can do these well, switch to Super Kegels. (See pages 64–65.) Tightening your pelvic floor muscles just before you stand up or sit down may make you more comfortable.
- Avoid constipation. Hard stools may slow the healing of hemorrhoids.

Q MY FRIEND SAID THE FIRST BOWEL MOVEMENT AFTER GIVING BIRTH IS REALLY SCARY. WHAT WOULD MAKE IT EASIER?

A Many women are uneasy about having that first bowel movement. Usually it's 2–3 days before there's a stool to pass. Although it may feel like your stitches might tear, they won't. Supporting your perineum with a wad of toilet paper may make you feel more secure. After the first bowel movement, the others aren't as scary. Eating high-fiber foods and drinking plenty of fluids will help prevent constipation. Your care provider may also prescribe a stool softener.

Q I PLAN TO FORMULA FEED. WHAT CAN I DO ABOUT FULL BREASTS?

A The birth of your baby signals your breasts to start making milk. It takes several days for the process to subside. Because more milk is produced when your breasts are emptied, don't stimulate them. Avoid the temptation to empty your breasts. If you pump milk out to make yourself more comfortable, you'll continue to produce milk and the discomfort will last longer. Instead, bind your breasts. You can wrap a wide Ace bandage around your chest several times. This should be snug but comfortable. Rewrap your breasts every couple of hours. You can also use cold packs to reduce swelling. Some women put cold cabbage leaves on their breasts. Showering may cause some of the milk to leak, making you a little more comfortable. You can also take pain relievers like ibuprofen or acetaminophen. These techniques work as well as medications to dry up milk, without the side effects.

Q I'M TOLD MY BELLY WILL LOOK REALLY BAD AFTER THE BABY IS BORN. HOW CAN I GET THINGS TONED UP?

A Lax muscles and stretched skin make a new mother's stomach sag and look lumpy. It'll take several months for your skin tone to return. Don't start abdominal exercises until you've talked to your care provider and checked your rectus muscles.

The rectus muscles are a pair of muscles that run from your pubic bone to your chest just to the right and left of center. During pregnancy these muscles can separate. After your baby is born, check if they've moved apart. Lie on your back with your knees bent and your feet flat on the floor. Lift your head and shoulders off the floor and feel just above your bellybutton. If there's a space of more than two fingers width, you'll need to do a special exercise. This time cross your arms over your belly and lift your head and shoulders as you exhale. Use your right hand to gently pull the left rectus muscle toward your bellybutton, and use your left hand to pull the right rectus muscle. Hold for about 5 seconds then lie back and relax for a minute. Do a set of four of these exercises a couple of times a day until the muscles are back in place. After that, you can do sit-backs, sit-ups, and other exercises to strengthen your abdominal muscles.

Q WHEN CAN I START AN EXERCISE ROUTINE?

A The timing will depend on how you feel and the advice of your care provider. Exercise like walking, swimming, and yoga can make you feel more energetic. However, don't overdo it. Your body will still be recovering from pregnancy and childbirth.

One way you can monitor if you're doing too much is to watch the color of your lochia. (See page 99.) As part of the healing process, lochia changes from red to brownish to yellowish. Once the lochia turns brownish, it shouldn't return to red, which indicates fresh blood. If the red does return, you need to rest more. Go to bed and rest until the red disappears. Then add activities more slowly.

Q WHEN WILL MY PARTNER AND I BE ABLE TO HAVE SEX AGAIN?

A For intercourse, it's best to wait at least four weeks until your tissues have healed and your lochia is no longer brown. The question then becomes, "When do *you* want to?" Some women are ready as soon as they can. Others aren't ready for months. Exhaustion, and the feeling that caring for the baby provides enough touching, can dampen sexual interest. You and your partner will need to talk about your desires.

Both of you may also be nervous about vaginal penetration, so take it slow. Using water-soluble lubrication such as K-Y jelly or Astroglide is helpful. A considerable number of women say they have some discomfort during sex for up to six months after the birth. If you have pain, report that to your care provider. The cause may be treatable.

Warning Signs to Call Your Care Provider

- Temperature over 101°F
- Vaginal bleeding that soaks one or more pads an hour
- Passing clots larger than a quarter
- Foul-smelling vaginal discharge
- Burning or pain when urinating
- Foul odor or pus coming from stitches or cesarean incision
- Red and painful spot on a breast or leg
- Any emotional warning signs listed on page 143

Q WHEN DO I NEED TO THINK ABOUT CONTRACEPTION?

A Get prepared before you have your baby. In order to prevent an unintended pregnancy, it's best to have protected sex from the beginning. You and your partner can use condoms and contraceptive foam or jelly. Women who formula feed often get a period seven to nine weeks after giving birth. However, the range is six weeks to six months. For breastfeeding women, it varies according to how frequently they nurse. The range is from six weeks to when the baby is weaned. Although frequent breastfeeding suppresses ovulation, it's not considered a reliable form of contraception. At your postpartum visit you and your care provider can determine your best option.

INFANT CARE

Q How do I find a healthcare provider for my baby?

A The process is similar to the one you used to choose your obstetrical care provider. (See pages 8–9.) First, determine the benefits and limitations of your health insurance. If you don't have insurance, many states have special programs for children's healthcare. Contact your city or county health department or search your state's Department of Health website.

If you'll have to pay for most of your baby's care, consider using community programs that provide low-cost immunizations and well-baby checkups. Your local health department can give you information about these programs. Usually these clinics don't see sick children. You'll need to use a walk-in clinic when your baby is ill if you don't have a care provider.

Pediatric care (the care for infants and children) is provided by several kinds of providers. (See the box below.) Determine which option suits your family. The advantage of having a pediatric care provider is that the person can be an ally and give you valuable advice about your baby's health and development. Therefore, you'll want to choose a person you trust. Meeting with the provider before you give birth is a good way to establish a relationship and get some of your baby-care questions answered.

Pediatric Care Options

- Pediatricians are physicians with special training related to infants and children. They see infants and children for scheduled checkups and when they're ill. A pediatrician can take care of your child through the teen years.
- Family practice physicians have had some training in pediatric care. They refer seriously ill children to pediatricians. The advantage of this option is that your whole family can see the same doctor. You may already be seeing this doctor for your regular or obstetrical care.
- Pediatric nurse practitioners are nurses with additional training in the care of infants and children. They refer to pediatricians if there's a complicated illness or problem. They may work in a clinic or with a pediatrician.

Q HOW DO I LOCATE A PEDIATRIC CARE PROVIDER?

A It's best to check with your health insurer first to see if there's a list of providers who are in their network. After that, gather recommendations from your obstetrical care provider, your childbirth educator or doula, and friends and family members who have children. When you get a referral, find out why the person likes that provider. Consider whether the reasons match your preferences. If you're giving birth in a hospital, you can get the names of the doctors who have privileges there. Then call the office or clinic to make sure the practice is taking new patients and accepts your insurance.

Questions about the Pediatric Practice

- What are the office hours?
- Are evening or Saturday appointments available?
- Is there an advice line or a time to call with questions that aren't urgent?
- How many providers are in the practice? How many are physicians? Nurse practitioners? Are there other services?
- What hospital(s) do they send patients to?
- Will someone from the practice see my baby in the hospital or birth center?
- How soon after discharge from the birth facility should my baby be seen in the office?
- When my baby is ill, how are these visits handled?
- What should I do if I have a medical concern when the office is closed?
- If I'm choosing a physician, does a nurse practitioner see my baby for some of the visits?

Q HOW DO I CHOOSE A PROVIDER FOR MY BABY?

A You'll want to know what services the office or clinic provides as well as some basic information, such as office hours. (See the box above.) Much of this information you can get over the phone. Many practices provide written materials that answer parents' most common questions.

Even more importantly, you'll want to know if you feel comfortable with the provider. This can best be decided in a face-to-face meeting. If at all possible, have your partner come, too. There may or may not be a charge for this visit. Ask about that when making the appointment. When you're waiting to see the provider, consider the following:

- How were you greeted when you arrived?
- How are the other parents and children treated by the staff?
- Is the waiting room designed with children in mind?
- Is there a separate entrance or waiting room for sick children?

The meeting with the provider is a time to ask any questions you have about baby-care issues including breastfeeding, circumcision, and immunizations. If you have a special family situation, you may want to discuss how this might affect your child's care. The provider is likely to ask you some questions about your pregnancy and medical history.

Q HOW CAN I GET MY PARTNER MORE INVOLVED WITH CAREGIVING TASKS?

A Parenting is a skill you learn by doing. A mother doesn't teach her partner how to parent. The baby does by responding to the parent's actions.

Before your baby is born, consider taking a parenting class that covers basic skills. That way you'll both know how to diaper, bathe, and dress your baby. Birth facilities and community education programs are likely to offer this type of class.

Whether you take a class or not, let your partner do the caregiving his or her own way. Your baby will be able to accommodate both of your styles. If your partner's way is not as smooth or efficient as yours, it's all right. This may be more a matter of having done it fewer times than being wrong. Avoid giving advice unless asked for it directly. If it's difficult for you to watch, leave the room.

If your community has Dad and Baby classes, suggest that your partner attend. These classes will give your partner an opportunity to get tips and support from other dads. It will also give you some time for yourself. Check your birth facility, community education bulletin, or local newspaper for class offerings. Information is also available at www.newdads.com.

ATTACHMENT

Q I HEAR DADS OFTEN FALL IN LOVE WITH THEIR BABY IMMEDIATELY. IF IT'S NOT LOVE AT FIRST SIGHT FOR ME, WILL THAT MEAN I LACK SOMETHING AS A MOTHER?

A Parents develop relationships with their babies on different timelines. Expectant mothers seem to be ahead of their partners in relating to the baby during pregnancy. That's because they experience the baby twenty-four hours a day. Partners, on the other hand, have an accumulating antici-

Infant Safety

- *Infant car seat.* Every time your baby is in a car, he must be in a safety seat approved for infants. The seat should be installed in the back seat so your baby is rear-facing. Never put your baby in the front seat if the vehicle has an active passenger-side airbag. Make sure the car seat is installed correctly. It shouldn't be able to slide or wiggle. Consider taking advantage of a community program that checks the installation of car seats. Contact your local police or health department, or find the nearest location online by visiting www.safekids.org.
- *Safe sleep.* When you put your baby in the crib or bassinette, put her on her back. This is the safest sleeping position because it lowers the risk of sudden infant death syndrome (SIDS). Make sure all of your baby's caregivers understand that babies should be put on their backs to sleep. For more information about SIDS, visit www.keepkidshealthy.com/welcome/safety/back_to_sleep.html.
- *Never shake a baby.* Babies' heads are large in proportion to their bodies, and their neck muscles are weak. Shaking a baby can cause severe brain damage and even death. Never ever shake a baby. If your baby's crying is frustrating you, put him gently in the crib on his back and walk out of the room. Give yourself a five-minute break. If you don't feel calm after that, call a friend or relative. Asking for help is a sign of strength. For more information about how to prevent shaking a baby, visit www.kidshealth.org/parent/medical/brain/shaken.html.
- *Never leave your baby alone in the bathtub.* Even a contoured baby tub isn't safe for her to be alone in. Set up the bath area with all that you'll need. Never leave your baby to get something or answer the phone.
- *Keep one hand on your baby at all times when using a changing table.* He can unexpectedly flip over and fall off. Arrange the area so the things you use are within reach. Put your baby in the crib when you need to clean up or wash your hands. Don't rely on a safety belt attached to the changing pad.

pation to see and touch the baby they've only been able to experience as movement inside the mother. When the baby is born, there's a climax of that anticipation. Many fathers and partners are immediately engrossed with the baby. They may be awed and overwhelmed by the strength of their feelings.

A mother has less available energy when the baby is born because she's had to birth the baby. In addition, she may still be focused on what's happening to her body. Even though the baby has been born, there's still more of the birth process going on, such as birthing the placenta. If the childbirth has been long or difficult, the mother may need some time to recover.

Many mothers say their feelings of love and attachment grow as they care for their baby. Through feeding, changing, bathing, and dressing their baby, they begin to feel the baby is truly theirs. It may take time to develop the bond between you and your baby, but it will happen and it will last a lifetime.

Q WE REALLY WANT A GIRL. UNLESS THE ULTRASOUND IS WRONG, WE'RE HAVING A BOY. WHAT IF I'M STILL DISAPPOINTED AFTER THE BABY IS BORN?

A Many expectant parents have a preference for a boy or girl. Usually this preference relates to feelings about boys and girls in general, such as boys are easier to raise. Parents, however, develop a relationship with a specific baby.

Although your disappointment about gender may not immediately disappear, it will likely fade. That's because after the birth you'll be able to see and hold your baby. Babies are powerful in their ability to draw parents—and others—to them. They invite you into interactions and respond to your actions. As you respond to and care for your baby, your attachment will grow. Soon it will be hard to imagine having any other baby.

POSTPARTUM EMOTIONS

Q WHAT'S THE DIFFERENCE BETWEEN BABY BLUES AND POSTPARTUM DEPRESSION?

A Baby blues appear a few days after birth and are usually over by two weeks post partum. Women have episodes of feeling teary or depressed, but these don't last long and resolve by themselves. Three in four mothers have episodes of baby blues.

Postpartum depression, on the other hand, often appears around the fourth week after birth or just prior to the beginning of a menstrual period. It can also appear after weaning or any time in the first year. It's characterized by having "good" days and "bad" days. Between 10 and 20 percent of mothers suffer from postpartum depression. New mothers can also have anxiety and/or panic disorder. Although postpartum depression may resolve on its own, it should not be ignored. Prolonged depression affects a baby's development. In addition, there may be a physical component that's caused by a thyroid condition. It's important to contact your care provider in order to get appropriate treatment.

If you're beginning to feel overwhelmed, taking a short break may make you feel better. Contact a friend or family member if:

- You're not able to sleep when your baby sleeps;
- You have significant changes in appetite;
- You feel more irritable or angry than usual;
- You wonder if you're a bad mother;
- You find it hard to make decisions.

Getting some support now may prevent further problems. If food, a nap, and a break from the responsibility of baby care don't make you feel better, contact your care provider.

Q IS POSTPARTUM DEPRESSION THE SAME AS POSTPARTUM PSYCHOSIS?

A No. These are two different problems. Postpartum psychosis is uncommon but a more severe problem. It comes on suddenly, often within three weeks after birth, and is evident within the first three months. Postpartum psychosis is persistent and severe, and may bring bizarre feelings and behavior. There's a danger of the woman hurting herself or her baby. This condition needs to be addressed immediately by a care provider. Tell your care provider or a responsible person if:

- You're experiencing anxiety or panic;
- You're afraid to be alone with your baby;
- You're worried about how you're feeling;
- You're afraid you might lose control;
- You're afraid of the thoughts you're having;
- You're having thoughts about hurting yourself;
- You can't tell your partner what you're feeling;
- There are other stressful events in your life;
- You're afraid to talk about how you're feeling, but you think someone should know.

Q I HAD A BOUT OF DEPRESSION BEFORE I GOT PREGNANT. DOES THAT MEAN I'M LIKELY TO GET POSTPARTUM DEPRESSION?

A Having depression before or during pregnancy increases the risk of postpartum depression. Make sure your care provider knows about your previous depression. It's important that you have support after your baby is born and that you have a way to get treatment immediately if the depression recurs. Remember, postpartum emotional disorders respond to treatment.

For more information about postpartum emotional disorders, see *This Isn't What I Expected: Overcoming Postpartum Depression* by Karen Kleiman and Valerie Raskin. You can also visit The Postpartum Stress Center at www.postpartumstress.com and Depression After Delivery, Inc. at www.depressionafterdelivery.com.

Q HOW CAN I LOWER MY RISK OF DEPRESSION?

A Factors that increase the risk of depression center around the lack of support. Cultures that have the lowest rate of postpartum depression have traditions that give a new mother lots of physical and emotional support for about a month after she gives birth. Things you can do include:

- Having a birth doula. Her support makes labor easier and improves satisfaction with the birth experience.
- Having a supportive partner. If your partner isn't able to be supportive, seek counseling before birth. Gather a support network that you can call upon after the baby is born.
- Having physical and emotional support. This will help you make the transition to being a confident mother.
- Minimizing outside responsibilities and stresses. Spending time and energy on other responsibilities reduces your resources for the work of post partum.

WHAT TO EXPECT RIGHT AFTER THE BIRTH

Q WHAT DO BABIES LOOK LIKE IN THE MOMENTS AFTER BIRTH?

A Before babies take their first breath, their skin color is dusky or bluish. Once a baby starts breathing, the skin becomes a more normal color. The hands and feet are the last to change. Because a newborn's skin is thin, you'll be able to see a lot of blood vessels. That means your baby may turn quite red when crying, or a mottled color when his skin gets cool. In the hours after birth, you may also notice marks or tiny bumps on his skin. Ask your nurse or care provider about them. Most of them disappear on their own.

Babies are wet when they're born. There may be streaks of bloody show from coming through the cervix. This usually gets wiped off when the baby is dried. There may also be traces of vernix (the creamy substance that protected the baby's skin in the womb). Any vernix that remains after the first bath can be rubbed into the baby's skin.

If your baby is born vaginally, his head may look a little misshaped. The bones of a baby's skull can slide over one another, making it easier for the baby to fit through the pelvis. His head will look rounder in a day or two. Some babies also have a soft lumpy bruise on the part of the head that was against the cervix in labor. This will disappear over the next several weeks. If forceps or a vacuum extractor was needed, your baby may show some bruising that will soon go away.

Your baby may have a lot of hair or just some fine down on his head. Many babies still have fine, downy hair called lanugo on their backs, shoulders, or ears. This will disappear within weeks. A newborn's breasts and genitals are enlarged because of the mother's hormones. These shrink to normal size within days. If you're concerned about anything you see, ask your nurse or care provider.

Q WHEN IS THE BEST TIME FOR THE UMBILICAL CORD TO BE CUT?

A There are several points of view about the timing. Some care providers cut the cord right after the baby is born. Others wait for the cord to stop pulsating. If the baby requires medical treatment or the cord is hampering the birth, the care provider may cut it as the baby is being born. Before the cord is cut, the care provider clamps it with two clamps. Then the cord between these clamps is cut with scissors. With a normal vaginal birth, the labor partner may be able to cut the cord. If this is important to you, discuss this with your care provider ahead of time.

Q WHAT DOES THE BABY'S APGAR SCORE MEAN?

A The Apgar score is a way to describe a baby's condition in the minutes after birth. It's an assessment of five things: heart rate, breathing, muscle tone, color, and reflex irritability. Each item is rated a 0, 1, or 2. The assessment is done at one minute and again at five minutes after birth. A score of 7 or better indicates the baby is in good condition. Scores of 6 or less usually indicate the baby needs medical attention. A baby rarely gets a 10 at the one-minute assessment. Normally the five-minute score is better than the one-minute score.

Q WHAT ELSE HAPPENS TO THE BABY RIGHT AFTER BIRTH?

A A baby needs to be dried and kept warm. Some providers place the baby on the mother's belly or chest right after birth and cover them both with a warm blanket. Other babies are taken to a nearby warmer. If you'd like your baby to stay with you, discuss this with your care provider ahead of time. Although babies are left naked for a while, they wear a cap to help their bodies retain heat.

Within the first hour, babies are given vitamin K to help with blood clotting, and an antibiotic ointment is put in their eyes. The baby is also weighed and measured. Because newborns are in a special quiet alert state for the first hour or so after birth, many parents ask that these procedures be delayed as long as possible or done at the mother's bedside.

Q WHAT'S SO SPECIAL ABOUT THIS FIRST HOUR AFTER BIRTH?

A For about the first hour after birth babies are usually in the quiet alert state. (See page 152.) They interact with their parents and nuzzle or suckle at the breast. This can be a very special time for parents as they begin to get to know their baby. At the same time babies get to see, smell, hear, and touch their parents. Babies who have been affected by pain medication given to their mothers may be less interactive and may appear sleepy.

Q WHAT HAPPENS IF I DON'T GET THIS SPECIAL TIME WITH MY BABY?

A If it isn't possible to spend the first hour after birth holding your baby, you can use other opportunities to hold and interact with her. Getting to know one another takes place over time. It isn't dependent on that first hour. One of the things you may want to consider for your birth plan is what your partner will do if your baby needs to go to a nursery immediately after birth.

Q I'VE RECEIVED INFORMATION ABOUT STORING MY BABY'S CORD BLOOD. WHAT THINGS SHOULD I CONSIDER?

A The blood in the baby's umbilical cord contains stem cells. These master cells can produce blood cells as well as immune system cells. They can be used instead of a bone marrow transplant as part of the treatment for some kinds of cancers and other diseases. In the future there may be other medical uses. Stem cells are a definite match for the baby and have a 1 in 4 chance of being a match for a sibling. If you have a family history of inherited disease, a genetic counselor can help you decide if this procedure might be beneficial. It's also a good idea to talk with your care provider.

The cord blood needs to be collected right after birth. The stem cells are then preserved by a special freezing process. Private companies provide these cryobanking services, which can be costly. There is an initial fee, often around $1,000, plus a yearly storage fee of about $100. You must register with the company ahead of time in order to receive a collection kit. Bring the kit to the birth facility so your nurse or care provider can collect the blood.

THE HOSPITAL STAY

Q WHAT WILL HAPPEN IN THE HOSPITAL?

A Soon after birth your nurse will put an identification tag on your baby's wrist and a second one on his ankle. You will also get an identification bracelet that has the same information as your baby's. Most hospitals have a fourth identification bracelet that's put on the other parent. That way your partner can get the baby from the nursery.

Your baby will be given a complete newborn exam. The person who does this exam will then talk to you about your baby. At that time ask any questions you may have about his health and appearance. Your baby will also get another exam before discharge.

Try to make the first appointment at the pediatric provider's office before you leave the hospital. This visit may be as soon as a day or two after discharge. Make sure to find out whom to call if you have questions about your baby's care after you leave the hospital or birth center.

Q WHAT KINDS OF THINGS WILL BE DONE FOR MY BABY WHILE WE'RE IN THE HOSPITAL?

A A nurse will monitor your baby's health, including checking your baby's heart rate, breathing, and temperature several times a day. In addition, your baby will be weighed once a day. It's normal for babies to lose up to 7 percent of their birth weight in the first two days. This is usually gained back before the end of the second week. You may be asked to keep a record of feedings and dirty diapers.

Most babies have a heel stick to get blood for tests that screen for inherited conditions that affect metabolism. Although these are rare, finding them early is very important. If you leave the hospital or birth center soon after giving birth, you'll need to have your baby tested by her care provider. Your baby's hearing may also be tested. This is usually done while she's sleeping. She may also be given the first in a series of vaccinations against hepatitis B.

Q HOW CAN I LEARN TO TAKE CARE OF MY BABY?

A Hospital stays after a vaginal birth are usually 48 hours, although some women choose to leave earlier. Women who give birth by cesarean usually stay 3–4 days. If you're still focused on trying to recover from the birth, this may feel too soon. If you've had opportunities to care for your baby, you're more likely to feel ready to go home.

Many postpartum areas are designed for babies to stay with their mothers. Staying together makes it easier to establish breastfeeding and to get to know your baby. Having your baby stay in your room as much as possible will help you get used to the sounds your baby makes and will enable your baby to feed whenever she's hungry. If you're unsure about any aspect of feeding your baby, ask for help. Consider having your partner or a family member stay with you. That may help you feel more comfortable having the baby stay in your room. That also gives your partner a chance to be involved in the baby's care. Ask your nurse to help you with anything you feel unsure of.

If your birth facility has babies stay in a nursery, ask that your baby be brought to you whenever she's hungry. If partners can't spend the night, suggest that your partner do as many of the caregiving tasks as possible when he or she is there.

Most hospitals give a bath demonstration or teach parents individually. Try to have your partner attend and be the one to bathe your baby. Some hospitals have a postnatal educator or nurse who does a class on newborns or talks with families individually about their babies. Take advantage of this opportunity to learn more about your baby and newborns in general.

A nurse can undress and dress a baby in no time. However, if it's your first couple of times, the task will take much longer. Ask for tips about getting the baby dressed, such as gently guiding the arm through the sleeve by reaching in from the wrist. Your nurse can also show you how to swaddle your baby. Swaddling (wrapping the baby snugly in a blanket) often reduces fussing because the baby feels more secure.

Q WE'RE HAVING A BOY. WHAT THINGS SHOULD WE CONSIDER ABOUT CIRCUMCISION?

A Circumcision is the removal of the skin around the end of the penis. If circumcision is not part of your religious or cultural tradition, the decision is a personal one. Here are some things to consider:

- Circumcision lowers the risk of a urinary tract infection during the baby's first year. Uncircumcised boys have a 1 percent chance of getting a urinary tract infection. Breastfeeding also lowers the risk of infection.
- If the foreskin of the penis becomes too tight, a circumcision will be needed in adulthood. At that time the recovery will be longer and more painful. This is a rare condition, however, and it's not necessary to routinely circumcise baby boys to prevent it.
- There may be a reduction in the risk of penile cancer if the penis is circumcised. This cancer is very rare. Good hygiene reduces the risk for uncircumcised men.
- If a boy is not circumcised, he will need to be taught how to pull back the foreskin to keep that area clean. This is very simple and easy for a boy to do.
- About 40 percent of boys in the United States are not circumcised, although rates vary by area. A circumcised boy will look like the other boys in the locker room. There will be other boys who are not circumcised.
- Some people think a boy's penis should look like his father's. In some families there's a difference between father and son or between brothers. These families say the difference is easy to explain.
- There's a small risk of damage to the penis during a circumcision. This risk is very low and most of the problems are minor.

- Circumcision is painful. Local anesthesia or other pain-reducing methods can be used.

If you want your son circumcised, you'll need to sign a consent form for this surgical procedure. Depending on your locality, your care provider or your baby's care provider will do the procedure. This is something you can discuss with your baby's care provider at your prenatal visit. (See pages 139–140.) To review the American Academy of Pediatrics statement on circumcision, go to http://aappolicy.aappublications.org/ and click on "Policy Statements."

YOUR NEWBORN'S SENSES

Q HOW WELL CAN BABIES HEAR RIGHT AFTER BIRTH?

A They hear well. As soon as fluid drains from their ears, they have normal hearing. Newborns prefer human voices to the sounds of objects. They like the sound of their mother's voice best. Babies also prefer higher pitched voices. That may be why adults usually pitch their voices higher when talking to a baby. Right from birth you'll be able to watch your baby turn toward sounds and familiar voices. She'll also enjoy lying on your chest and listening to your heartbeat.

Q HOW WELL CAN BABIES SEE AT BIRTH?

A Sight is the least developed sense at birth. Newborns see things best when they're about 7–10 inches away. This is roughly the distance to a parent's face when the baby is cradled in the parent's arms. Babies can see up to 18 inches away, but not very clearly. In the beginning, dimming the lights may make it easier for your baby to keep his eyes open.

Babies like to look at faces best. They concentrate on the mouth and eyes—the areas that have the greatest contrast. When you hold your baby, you'll notice that he studies your face. He's getting to know what you look like. Babies remember what they see. Your baby will notice if you look different at some point, such as wearing glasses when you normally don't. Babies look longer at something that's unfamiliar.

Q WILL MY BABY REALLY MIMIC ME AND STICK OUT HER TONGUE?

A In the quiet alert state babies may mimic a parent's expression. Two of the easiest things to do are to form an O with your lips or stick out your tongue. After watching you do it, your baby may, too. You may not notice that she mimics your other expressions, such as lip pursing and frowns. Without thinking about it, you'll mimic your baby's expressions. This interplay is part of what makes looking at your baby so captivating.

Interacting with Your Baby

- Create a calm environment.
- Watch for signs that your baby is ready to interact.
- Help your baby maintain a quiet alert state.
- Respect your baby's signals for a time out.
- Be sensitive to your baby's temperament.

Q WHAT ABOUT A NEWBORN'S SENSE OF SMELL?

A Right from birth newborns demonstrate an excellent sense of smell. By the time they're two days old, babies can identify the smell of their mother's milk on a breast pad. Mothers can also identify their baby by scent.

STATES

Q WHY IS IT HELPFUL TO KNOW ABOUT A NEWBORN'S SLEEP STATES?

A Understanding the difference between quiet sleep and active sleep can make parenting a little easier. Newborns have irregular sleep periods that last between 50 minutes and several hours. During this time they cycle through quiet sleep and active sleep. In quiet sleep they're still and have rhythmic breathing. They usually remain in this state for only 20–30 minutes at a time. It's hard to waken them from quiet sleep. If you need to waken your baby for a feeding, it's best to wait until he moves into active sleep.

When babies are in active sleep, their breathing is irregular. They may squirm, twitch, and make faces as well as sucking motions. Sometimes when parents see their baby in active sleep, they think their baby is awake and needs them. Make sure your baby really is awake and signaling for your attention. If your baby is in active sleep and is left undisturbed, he may remain asleep for a bit longer.

Q SOMETIMES MY BABY SLEEPS THROUGH FAMILY AND FRIENDS COMING TO SEE HER. THEN, WHEN THEY'VE GONE, SHE WAKES UP. WHY IS THAT?

A When the environment gets overstimulating, babies sometimes fall asleep so they don't have to interact. They use sleep in a protective way. Try to limit activity around your baby when you have visitors. Don't pick her up or try to coax her into alertness. Instead, keep the lights low and talk quietly. Your baby may then come out of her guarded sleep. As your baby gets older, she'll be more willing to interact.

Q AT TIMES MY BABY SEEMS TO BE AWAKE, BUT HE ISN'T VERY RESPONSIVE. WHAT SHOULD I DO?

A There is a transitional, drowsy state between sleeping and being awake. In this state your baby's eyes will be dull and unfocused, opening and closing sleepily. He may wriggle and whimper but won't have purposeful movements. How you respond depends on what you want to happen. If you're trying to get him to go to sleep, avoid stimulating him. If you want him to wake up, pick him up and talk to him. You can also give him something to look at. That will help him move into an alert state.

Q WHAT'S THE DIFFERENCE BETWEEN THE QUIET ALERT AND ACTIVE ALERT STATES?

A Babies are available for play and interaction in the quiet alert state. At this time they're calm and attentive. Your baby may be able to stay in this state longer by sucking on a finger or pacifier. Your talking softly may also help. As your baby's nervous system matures, her quiet alert periods will get longer.

In the active alert state babies breathe more irregularly. They can no longer stay focused and have less control over their movements. These are signs that they may be getting hungry or need to rest. If their need isn't met, babies usually start fussing or crying.

Q MY BABY LOOKS AT ME INTENTLY FOR A SHORT TIME AND THEN LOOKS AWAY. IS HE BORED?

A No, your baby is just taking a short break. New babies can only maintain their intent focus for short periods of time. Then they need a little rest. They signal this by looking or moving away. (See page 153.) If that doesn't work, they show signs of distress.

When your baby signals for a time out, respond by stopping your activity and softening your focus. Avoid looking directly at him until he invites you back. When he's ready to interact again, he'll look at you and brighten his face or widen his eyes. He may also move his arms or legs to catch your attention. Following your baby's lead allows you to interact with him for a longer period of time. Over the next several months your baby's ability to maintain focus will gradually increase.

Q IS CRYING ANOTHER BABY STATE?

A Yes, crying is the most aroused state. Crying signals that the baby needs something. Babies have different kinds of cries for different needs. These include being uncomfortable, hungry, tired, bored, ill, or needing to discharge tension. Parents learn what their baby's different cries mean by trying different things and seeing how their baby responds. This, however, takes time. In the weeks after birth parents get better at interpreting their baby's cries, and babies get better at signaling what they need.

Q ISN'T CRYING A SIGN THAT BABIES ARE HUNGRY?

A The most common reason for newborns to cry is hunger. However, crying is a late sign of hunger. Babies are easier to feed before they get worked up by crying. Earlier cues for hunger include:
- Sucking;
- Smacking their lips;
- Mouthing their hand;
- Rooting (opening their mouth and turning toward the cheek that has been touched);
- Bobbing their head on their mother's chest.

Ways That Babies Signal the Need for a Time Out

- Looking away
- Turning their head
- Arching their back
- Fussing
- Breathing faster or harder
- Briefly holding their breath
- Getting pale, red, or mottled
- Startling
- Sneezing or coughing
- Hiccupping
- Spitting up
- Having a bowel movement

DEVELOPING A RELATIONSHIP WITH YOUR BABY

Q WHY IS TOUCHING A BABY SO IMPORTANT?

A Babies are sensitive to touch and are nurtured by it. This includes skin-to-skin feeding, infant massage, and cuddling. Activities like bathing, diapering, and dressing are opportunities to nurture your baby through touch. At first most babies don't like to be bathed or changed. However, within weeks many enjoy these activities.

Caregiving is also play time. Your voice and eye contact, along with your touch, turn a routine interaction into a wonderful exchange. Caregiving strengthens your relationship with your baby.

Q HOW SOON CAN I TELL WHAT MY BABY IS LIKE?

A Temperament describes how a person responds to the world. There are some clues to temperament even before birth, such as how sensitive the baby is to sounds and the baby's activity level. As soon as they're born, you can see differences between babies. For example, some babies cry a lot in the minutes immediately after birth. A few even seem to be protesting. Other babies cry very little. Some look around or listen intently to the voices and sounds around them. Over time parents realize that aspects of their child's temperament were apparent from birth.

You may not be able to determine aspects of your baby's temperament right away. Some babies need a few days to recover from the birth process. Until then they seem sleepy and not very responsive. Gentle handling and holding them skin-to-skin will help them recover. Then, you'll be able to see more of your baby's personality.

Q WHY IS A BABY'S TEMPERAMENT IMPORTANT?

A Temperament shapes a baby's response to soothing and handling. That influences how parents and others interact with the baby. For example, some newborns are wonderful cuddlers. They immediately snuggle up against your neck, their bodies conforming to the shape of your chest and shoulder. Others don't want to cuddle. They prefer to be held so they're turned toward the world. In addition, newborns have preferences about movement and rocking.

Temperament also affects a baby's sensitivity to temperature and discomfort, the response to hunger, the need for sleep, the amount of crying, and the amount of stimulation they can handle. That makes some babies seem "easy" while others are more difficult. As a result, your baby's temperament can affect your confidence in your ability to parent. For more information about newborns, read *Your Amazing Newborn* by Marshall and Phyllis Klaus.

CONSIDERATIONS

Q WHAT MAKES BREASTFEEDING EASY?

A Although during the first couple of weeks you may feel awkward while breastfeeding, you and your baby will soon become skilled at it. After that, breastfeeding is easy because your body takes care of feeding your baby. You don't have to worry about buying and mixing formula or washing and filling bottles. All you have to do is offer your breast. In addition, you and your baby will enjoy breastfeeding because it makes both of you feel good. Your baby has the warmth and security of being held close to feed. You get the relaxation and sense of well-being that breastfeeding hormones create.

Q WHAT MAKES BREASTFEEDING HARD?

A Even though breastfeeding is natural, it's a skill that needs to be mastered over the first weeks after birth. Some babies are avid feeders right from the start. Others need time and patience. This is especially true for babies whose nervous systems have been affected by childbirth pain medication or who have had a difficult birth.

Our society also makes breastfeeding difficult. Hospital procedures that separate mothers and babies discourage breastfeeding. In some areas there's opposition to breastfeeding in public. That may put a burden on you to find a private place to feed your baby. Family and friends may question your decision to breastfeed and worry aloud that your baby isn't getting enough milk. That may raise your doubts and concerns. If you don't have support, you may feel frustrated and discouraged.

You can make breastfeeding easier by identifying your support people before your baby is born. Also, find someone who's knowledgeable about breastfeeding and can help you address your concerns. Not getting help in the beginning can turn a small problem into a much bigger one.

Q HOW CAN I GET BREASTFEEDING SUPPORT?

A Breastfeeding support can come from a variety of sources. Check them out while you're still pregnant.

- Your care provider or birth facility may offer breastfeeding classes. You and your partner will be able to learn things that will help make the first weeks of breastfeeding easier.
- Ask if your hospital is certified as Baby Friendly. These hospitals follow ten steps that help women breastfeed their babies.
- Peer support is available through organizations like La Leche League. Trained leaders offer both individual counseling and meetings that are designed for pregnant women and nursing mothers. You can get information before and after your baby is born as well as meet other breastfeeding mothers. Look up La Leche League in your phone book or visit www.lalecheleague.org.
- Lactation consultants are experts trained and certified by an international organization. They provide individual counseling. Some lactation consultants are on staff at a birth facility, clinic, or care provider's office. Others are in private practice. Some see mothers before they're discharged from the birth facility, and then are available by phone, on an outpatient basis, or as part of an office visit. Contact your hospital or birth center to see what services will be available for you. Private consultants usually come to your home. Your birth facility, care provider, or childbirth educator may be able to provide a list of private lactation consultants. In addition, you can look in the phone book under "breastfeeding" or "lactation," or visit www.ilca.org/find/index.php.
- Birth doulas and postpartum doulas often provide information and support. If you're using a doula, ask her what she does and if she has training and certification.
- Family members and friends who have breastfed can support your decision to breastfeed and share tips from their experiences.
- It may also be helpful to have a breastfeeding book such as *Amy Spangler's Breastfeeding: A Parent's Guide* or La Leche League's *Womanly Art of Breastfeeding*.

Q MY PARTNER WANTS TO BE INVOLVED IN FEEDING THE BABY. HOW CAN I DO THAT IF I BREASTFEED?

A Feeding the baby is often a focus of activity because it's central to survival. Right from the start your partner can provide another essential element: nurturing the baby through touch. Touching and stroking a baby promotes brain development as well as attachment. All babies need this kind of nurturance. Your partner's lightly stroking the baby will stimulate a sense of well-being in both of them. For more information on infant massage see www.infantmassage.com.

In addition, if your baby needs your expressed milk, your partner can be involved in those feedings. Most breastfeeding experts recommend waiting to introduce a bottle until the baby is suckling well. Until then, your partner can use a medicine spoon, dropper, or infant feeding cup.

BENEFITS

Q ARE BREASTFED BABIES REALLY HEALTHIER THAN FORMULA-FED BABIES?

A Yes, breastfed babies are healthier. Formula-fed babies have more urinary tract, respiratory, and ear infections. They also have more diarrhea and colic. Formula feeding increases the risk of some childhood cancers and may increase the risk of sudden infant death syndrome (SIDS). Breastfeeding health benefits are long lasting. Formula feeding increases the risk for food allergies, asthma, insulin-dependent diabetes, and chronic bowel diseases. It may cause a tendency toward higher cholesterol levels and higher blood pressure. Formula-fed children are also more likely to be overweight.

Q I'VE HEARD THAT BREASTFED BABIES ARE SMARTER. IS THAT TRUE?

A Children who were breastfed score higher on IQ tests than formula-fed children. This is especially true of children who were born prematurely. Breast milk is perfectly suited for a baby's optimal growth and promotes nervous system development and brain growth.

Q IF I BREASTFEED WILL I LOSE WEIGHT FASTER AFTER MY BABY IS BORN?

A Breastfeeding helps you steadily lose weight because producing breast milk requires calories. Breastfeeding draws on the fat stores your body created in pregnancy. A safe rate of weight loss is about a pound a week. However, breastfeeding also increases appetite. It's important to continue making healthy food choices. (See pages 14–17.)

Q ARE THERE OTHER HEALTH BENEFITS FOR THE MOTHER?

A Right from the baby's birth there are health benefits from breastfeeding. The baby suckling at the breast causes the mother's uterus to contract, which prevents excessive bleeding (postpartum hemorrhage) and helps the uterus heal faster. There are also long-term health benefits, especially for women who breastfeed for a year or more, including a lower risk of breast, ovarian, and uterine cancers and fewer hip fractures because of increased bone density.

PREPARATION

Q WHAT DO I NEED TO DO TO PREPARE MY BREASTS FOR BREASTFEEDING?

A There's very little you need to do. Throughout pregnancy keep your breasts clean by washing them with water once a day. You don't need to put lotion or creams on your nipples. The Montgomery glands, those bumps on the areola (the area around the nipple), lubricate and disinfect them. You don't need to do anything to toughen your nipples.

You may or may not see colostrum leak from your nipples during pregnancy. Colostrum is your "first milk," the golden milk your breasts produce toward the middle of pregnancy. Avoid expressing this colostrum. Your baby needs it after birth. In addition, expressing could cause uterine contractions that lead to premature labor.

Q I THINK I HAVE FLAT NIPPLES. WHAT SHOULD I DO?

A Nipples come in all shapes and sizes, and they all work. When most women gently pinch the skin at the base of the nipple, the nipple comes forward or protrudes. For some women, however, the nipple remains flat or even tucks in (inverts). Nipples that are flat or inverted sometimes make it harder for the baby to latch on.

If you're still in early pregnancy, pregnancy changes may take care of the problem. If not, you can consult a lactation consultant about the best option for you. One option is to wait until the baby is born. Some babies latch on easily to any type of nipple. If your baby has trouble latching on, try using a breast pump just before nursing. That will make the nipple protrude, making it easier for your baby to latch on. Another option is to wear breast shells inside your bra during the last weeks of pregnancy and between feedings until your baby latches on easily. These shells press on the areolas and help the nipples protrude. After a few weeks of nursing, your baby will be able to latch on well without your doing these things.

Q WHAT EQUIPMENT SHOULD I HAVE ON HAND?

A You don't need any equipment to breastfeed. However, you may want to have some supplies on hand.

Most women are more comfortable wearing a nursing bra that has flaps that open and allow you to easily and discreetly nurse your baby. These bras come in a variety of styles. You may find it helpful to buy your first bra at a maternity or specialty store that has experience fitting nursing bras. A bra that fits in the last weeks of pregnancy will usually fit during the early weeks after birth. You don't need to wear a bra at night if you're more comfortable without one.

You may want to have a supply of breast pads on hand. These small pads are worn inside the bra to absorb leaking breast milk. Don't buy pads that have a plastic lining. These trap moisture and can cause sore nipples. If you're planning to store breast milk, you'll need a supply of collection bags or containers.

Q WILL I NEED A BREAST PUMP? IF SO, WHAT KIND?

A Not every mother needs a breast pump. You need one only if you plan to be away from your baby at times you would normally be nursing. You can hand express milk to give to your baby or to occasionally soften an overly full breast. However, if you're going to be expressing your milk regularly, it's more efficient to use a breast pump.

There are several types of pumps. Which one is best depends on how often you're going to use it. If you're planning to store breast milk to be given to your baby while you're at work or school, an electric pump is best. It's also the best choice if you need to maintain your milk supply while your baby is being fed breast milk from a spoon or bottle. Electric pumps can be rented or purchased.

A battery powered pump or hand pump may work well if you're only going to pump occasionally. Pumps vary greatly in quality and effectiveness. Consider talking with a lactation consultant to determine the type and style that's best for you. You can often see and learn about different types of pumps at a breastfeeding class.

CONCERNS

Q DO I HAVE TO EAT A SPECIAL DIET WHEN I'M BREASTFEEDING?

A Breastfeeding does not require any specific diet. Most women can eat the foods they want. Some babies get fussy after the mother eats a particular food, especially if she eats a lot of it. If that seems to be happening to your baby, eliminate the food and see if this makes a difference. Sometimes a baby will reject a nursing after the mother has eaten a strongly flavored meal. You don't have to limit yourself to bland foods, however. Your baby has already been introduced to the flavors of your diet through swallowing amniotic fluid.

Q CAN I DRINK ALCOHOL WHILE I'M NURSING?

A Alcohol passes into breast milk, so your baby will be exposed to alcohol when you drink. A mother who has three or more drinks a day will affect her baby's brain development. It's best, therefore, to avoid drinking alcohol regularly. If you have an occasional serving of alcohol, breastfeed your baby before having the drink. Then wait at least two hours before breastfeeding.

Q I SMOKE CIGARETTES. DOES THAT MEAN I SHOULDN'T BREASTFEED?

A Because of the many benefits of breast milk, it's better to breastfeed even if you smoke. Whether the mother breastfeeds or not, a mother's smoking increases the number of the baby's respiratory illnesses and ear infections and increases the risk of sudden infant death syndrome (SIDS). Smoking may decrease milk production. If you can't stop smoking, limit the number of cigarettes to as few as possible. In addition, limit your baby's exposure to the harmful effects of secondhand smoke. Don't smoke around your baby and ask others not to.

Q I'VE HEARD BREAST MILK CONTAINS PCBs AND OTHER TOXINS. ISN'T THAT A REASON NOT TO BREASTFEED?

A News articles may make it sound like breast milk is the source of the harmful chemical. However, when toxins are found in breast milk, it means that the environment contains these chemicals. Everyone is being exposed to them. It's still better to breastfeed your baby because of the numerous health benefits of breast milk.

Q WILL BREASTFEEDING CAUSE MY BREASTS TO SAG?

A Breastfeeding doesn't damage breast tissue. In fact, breastfeeding is beneficial because it reduces the risk of breast cancer. Whether breasts sag is related to genetics, weight, and breast changes that occur during pregnancy. Wearing a well-fitting bra during pregnancy and breastfeeding may make you more comfortable. However, you don't have to always wear a bra. Do what's most comfortable for you. If you prefer an underwire bra, choose a well-fitting one. If the wire presses into your breast tissue, it can cause plugged ducts and breast infections.

YOUR MILK SUPPLY

Q HOW CAN I TELL IF MY BABY IS GETTING ENOUGH MILK?

A Although you can't measure the amount of milk going in, there are several ways you can be assured that your baby is feeding well. During the first month, breastfeed whenever your baby gives hunger cues such as rooting, licking, sucking, or putting her hand to her mouth. Your baby needs to feed about every one to three hours. That means at least eight to twelve feedings each twenty-four hours. After each feeding, she should seem satisfied. During the first month or so, she should have at least four good-sized stools (at least the size of a quarter) each twenty-four hours. This soiling can look like a yellow stain or a mixture of mustard and cottage cheese. She should also have at least six wet diapers a day. Disposable diapers can make it difficult to determine if your

Breastfeeding Tips

- Nurse frequently (eight to twelve times in twenty-four hours).
- Let your baby nurse on one side for as long as she wants.
- Offer the second breast after burping her.
- Alternate the breast that's offered first.
- If necessary, hand express a little milk to soften the area around the nipple. That may help her get a better latch.
- Make sure your baby has a good latch.
- Use several nursing positions each day.

baby has urinated. If this is the case, put a strip of facial tissue between her bottom and the diaper.

Another sign that your baby is getting milk is that you can hear her swallow. At the beginning of the feeding, you may hear only sucking. This triggers the let-down reflex, making your milk start to flow. After that you can hear or see your baby swallow as well as suck. Active swallowing means swallowing with nearly every suck. Most newborns need to actively swallow for at least 10–20 minutes in a feeding. Toward the end of a feeding, after your baby has swallowed regularly, she'll suck several times or more between swallows.

Signs that she has ended the feeding include sleeping, being quietly awake, or no longer giving hunger cues. When the feeding is over, your breast will feel softer. Look for your baby to gain 4–8 ounces a week after the first or second week. Babies usually double their birth weight in four to six months and triple it in a year.

Q CAN I GIVE MY NEWBORN A PACIFIER IF I'M BREASTFEEDING?

A In the early weeks it's usually best not to give a baby a pacifier until you've gotten breastfeeding established. Sucking on a pacifier can delay your baby's feeding. It's the frequent feeding that builds up your milk supply. Babies need to develop good suckling (mouth and tongue movements used for breastfeeding). A pacifier can prolong poor sucking habits, making your nipples sore. If your baby is fussy and doesn't want to nurse, consider offering a clean finger (fingernail side down) for your baby to suck on. Some babies, however, suckle well and have a great need to suck. They're able to use a pacifier to meet some of that sucking need.

Q WHEN CAN BOTTLES BE INTRODUCED?

A This will depend on you and your baby. As with the pacifier, it's best not to introduce a bottle nipple until your baby is suckling well. That way your baby won't start to prefer the bottle to the breast. If your partner wants to feed your baby before this time, give your breast milk from a medicine spoon or dropper.

It's best not to use a bottle with formula or water for the first four weeks. The supply of breast milk is related to demand. You'll need this time for your body to build up a good milk supply.

Usually by six to twelve weeks breastfeeding is well established. Then you'll be able to use bottles for the times when you aren't available. Pumping after some nursings will provide breast milk you can store. If you don't have stored breast milk, you can substitute formula. However, the key to a good milk supply is to nurse whenever possible. Your baby's suckling will get your breasts to produce more milk than even the best breast pumps.

PROBLEM SOLVING

Q WHAT CAN I DO IF MY BABY HAS TROUBLE LATCHING ON AFTER BIRTH?

A Some babies need time to recover after birth. They may be sleepy, fussy, or have uncoordinated suckling. You can help your baby adapt to life outside the womb by providing a lot of skin-to-skin contact. This closeness reduces stress and helps your baby learn to breastfeed. All you have to do is hold your baby to your bare chest. He should wear only a diaper and perhaps a cap. Keep his back covered with a receiving blanket. Gently offer your breast when you notice any hunger cues. (See page 153.) This gives him frequent opportunities to nuzzle, lick, root, and learn to latch on. Your partner can also spend time holding him skin-to-skin, returning him to you when there are hunger cues.

If several hours pass and your baby hasn't latched, you may want to begin expressing colostrum. You can hand express or use a pump. Offer him this colostrum from a spoon, cup, or dropper until he begins nursing well. If he hasn't begun nursing by the time you're to be discharged, contact a lactation consultant for help.

Getting Your Baby Latched On Well

- Keep your baby's head, shoulder, and hip in a straight line.
- Hold your breast so you can guide it, but don't distort the shape of your nipple.
- Tickle your baby's cheek so he turns toward the breast.
- Tickle your baby's lips with your nipple. When his mouth opens wide, bring the baby to your breast. Avoid leaning forward and bringing your breast to your baby.
- Both the nipple and much of the areola should be in his mouth. His lips should be forward and not curled over the gum.
- Your baby's chin, cheeks, and the tip of his nose should touch your breast.
- If your baby hasn't latched on well, break the suction, remove him from your breast, and start again.

Q HOW CAN I PREVENT SORE NIPPLES?

A In the early weeks of breastfeeding, you may experience some soreness for about the first minute after your baby latches on. If this doesn't disappear, it's best to get her off the breast and start over. To get your baby to release the nipple, slide your finger inside her cheek or press on your breast near her mouth. This will break the suction, allowing her mouth to slide off the nipple rather than pulling on it.

It's important that your baby latches on correctly. (See page 163.) In addition, the suggestions on page 161 will help prevent sore nipples.

Q I HAVE SORE NIPPLES. WHAT SHOULD I DO?

A Focus on speeding the healing process and making sure the baby has a good latch:
• Speed healing by applying a little breast milk or colostrum to your nipples after your baby has finished nursing.
• Expose your breasts to the air to make sure they dry. Trapped moisture increases soreness.
• Lansinoh (purified lanolin) may help heal cracked nipples.
• Start nursing on the less sore side. If milk begins to leak out of the sore side, it's a good time to switch to it.
• Give the sore nipple a rest by pumping for a few feedings or even a day.
• If you can't determine what's causing the poor latch, seek help. A lactation consultant or breastfeeding expert can give you information and support to solve the problem.

Q HOW CAN I PREVENT ENGORGEMENT?

A When your milk comes in, your breasts will likely get full and tender. Additional blood flow adds to this swelling, which can make it difficult for your baby to latch on to the nipple. The suggestions in the Breastfeeding Tips box (page 161) are useful in minimizing this swelling. In addition, try the following:
• Gently massage your breasts to increase circulation to get rid of the extra fluid.

- Get into a shower and let the warm water flow over your breasts. This may help get the milk flowing.
- Another way to get milk flowing is to apply warmed rice socks or a warmed towel to your breasts.
- If your baby doesn't suckle both breasts, hand express or pump some milk from the second breast to reduce fullness.
- After breastfeeding, apply a soft ice pack or a bag of frozen peas to your breasts to ease soreness. Wrap these in a towel to prevent skin damage. Some women use cold cabbage leaves. Use a cold pack or cabbage leaves before breastfeeding if the breast is so full your baby is having trouble latching on.
- Consider taking ibuprofen to decrease the inflammation and increase your comfort.
- If the swelling hasn't decreased after twenty-four hours, or if your baby is unable to latch on due to overfull breasts, seek advice from a lactation consultant or breastfeeding expert.

Q HOW CAN I PREVENT LEAKING BREASTS?

A During the first month or so of breastfeeding, it's common for breasts to leak. Sometimes when the milk lets down in the suckled breast, the other breast begins flowing. To prevent this leaking, press the heel of your hand into your nipple. Pinching the nipple also works but is less discreet. Most women find that the leaking diminishes after breastfeeding has gotten well established.

Sometimes leaking is a reminder that it's been a while since you last nursed. Leaking can happen when your baby is feeding irregularly or skips a feeding, resulting in overfull breasts. If you can, stop and nurse your baby.

Your breasts may also leak if you think about or hear your baby. It can even happen when you hear another baby cry. Crossing your arms firmly across your breasts will stop the flow of milk. However, frequently applying pressure to your breasts to stop leaking may cause a plugged duct or a breast infection.

Your breasts are also likely to leak, even spray, when you're sexually aroused. Nursing your baby before having intimate time with your partner will minimize this and give you more time together.

SPECIAL CIRCUMSTANCES

Q CAN I BREASTFEED IF I HAVE A CESAREAN BIRTH?

A Yes. Having a cesarean birth doesn't affect your ability to breastfeed. The pain medication you'll get is safe for your baby. If you've had spinal or epidural anesthesia, you may be able to nurse in the recovery room. Talk to your care provider about including this in your birth plan.

Ask a breastfeeding expert for suggestions related to comfortable feeding positions and other post-cesarean tips. Take advantage of all offers of household help so you can devote your energy to breastfeeding and being with your baby.

Q I'M EXPECTING TWINS. HOW CAN I BREASTFEED BOTH OF THEM?

A Your body will produce the amount of milk your babies need. The more your babies nurse, the more milk you'll produce. Eating well and drinking plenty of fluids will give your body what it needs to feed your babies. It may be easier to start out nursing one baby at a time so you can make sure that baby is nursing well. After a while you may find it more efficient to nurse both babies at the same time. You can also pump and give the breast milk in a bottle or cup when breastfeeding is not possible. Consider getting support from a breastfeeding expert and from other mothers who have nursed multiples. For more help, read *Mothering Multiples: Breastfeeding and Caring for Twins or More* by Karen Gromada.

Q I NEED TO GO BACK TO WORK SOON AFTER THE BABY IS BORN. IS IT WORTH IT TO BREASTFEED FOR ONLY A FEW WEEKS?

A Yes. However long you breastfeed will benefit your baby. The colostrum she'll get right after birth will help her pass meconium, the first bowel movement. Colostrum is also rich in antibodies. As your milk comes in, the transition to mature milk will help her intestines adjust to digesting milk.

If breastfeeding is well established before you have to return to work, you may choose to continue nursing for some of the feedings. Pumping and leaving a supply of breast milk may also be an option. A lactation consultant can help you establish a breastfeeding and work pattern or plan a weaning process.

CONSIDERATIONS

Q WHAT MAKES FORMULA FEEDING EASY?

A People other than the mother can feed the baby. This may be important if the mother is going to be away from her baby for periods of
time. It may also allow the mother to get more rest by involving other family members in the feeding process. It's socially acceptable to bottle-feed a
baby in public, so parents don't need to find a private place to feed their
baby. Mothers who have been advised by their care provider not to breastfeed for medical reasons can formula feed their baby.

Q WHAT MAKES FORMULA FEEDING HARD?

A Several reasons:
• It takes time and may be inconvenient to clean and prepare bottles.
• Formula must be measured carefully and prepared according to instructions.
• If there's any question about the safety of the water, it must be boiled
  before it's used to prepare the formula.
• You can only mix one day's supply. Even formula stored in the refrigera-
  tor should be discarded after twenty-four hours.
• You have to plan ahead and bring a bottle with you if you're going out
  with your baby.
• If your baby has problems digesting the formula, it may take time to find
  the best formula for your baby.
• Formula is an added expense ($1,000 or more for the first year).

PREPARATION

Q WHAT EQUIPMENT AND SUPPLIES SHOULD I HAVE ON HAND?

A You'll need a supply of bottles. These can be made of glass or plastic.
They come in four-ounce and eight-ounce sizes. A new baby drinks
about 2 ounces at a feeding, so the smaller size is fine for a while. If you
use plastic bottles, throw them out when they begin to cloud. This is a sign
that the plastic is beginning to break down. A newborn feeds a minimum of

eight times in a twenty-four-hour period and needs a new bottle each time. The common recommendation is to have six to eight bottles on hand. Another option is to use a "soft bottle" system that has disposable plastic liners.

You'll also need a supply of nipples. Nipples come in a variety of styles. You can choose one and have your baby get used to that choice. Or, you can buy a few different styles and see which one your baby likes best. If you're going to use a pacifier, have it be the same style as the nipple.

You'll need a way to clean the bottles and nipples. Many families who own dishwashers wash the bottles and nipples with their regular dishes. You can buy a special basket to hold the nipples, collars, and caps. You can also wash the bottles and nipples in hot soapy water and let them air dry. A bottle brush and a nipple brush will make the cleaning easier. It's usually not necessary to sterilize the bottles and nipples. However, if that's something you want or need to do, you can buy a bottle sterilizer.

Finally, you'll need formula and a way to measure and mix it. A glass measuring cup will help you measure the correct amount of water. You can also use it to heat water in the microwave. Powdered formula containers include a measuring scoop.

Q WHAT KIND OF FORMULA IS BEST?

A That depends on your baby and your preferences. Pediatric care providers recommend that the formula be iron-fortified. Only babies with a rare medical condition should drink formula that isn't iron-fortified. Most babies do well on a formula made from cow's milk. If your baby has trouble digesting milk sugars, there are lactose-free formulas and soy-based formulas. You might also choose a soy-based formula if you don't want your baby to have animal products. In addition, there are hypoallergenic formulas. Your baby's care provider can help you with the best choice for your baby.

Formula comes in three forms: ready-to-feed, concentrate, and powdered. Ready-to-feed is the most expensive and most convenient. Concentrate comes in a can and must be mixed with water. It's less expensive than ready-to-feed. Powdered formula is the most economical and is mixed with water. It comes in various-size containers and individual packets. When mixing formula, it's very important to follow the directions exactly. Adding additional formula or additional water will be harmful to your baby.

Babies need to drink formula for the first year. Do not use evaporated milk or regular, low-fat, or skim milk. These do not have all the nutrients your baby needs. They're also harder for your baby to digest. In addition, don't dip the nipple in honey or add honey to your baby's formula. Babies under a year can be poisoned by infant botulism.

FEEDING FUNDAMENTALS

Q SHOULD I WARM THE BOTTLE?

A Often young babies prefer a bottle that's warmed to body temperature. As they get older, babies usually accept or even prefer a cooler temperature. Some babies don't seem to care about the temperature. Follow your baby's preference.

Q WHY SHOULDN'T I HEAT A BOTTLE IN THE MICROWAVE?

A A microwave doesn't heat evenly. This can result in your baby getting some formula that's hotter than you intended. Hot liquid can burn your baby's esophagus. If the bottle is already made, you can warm it in hot water that comes from the faucet. If you're mixing powdered formula, you can warm the water in the microwave. The stirring or shaking needed to dissolve the powder will equalize the temperature. Always check the temperature of the formula in the bottle before you begin a feeding.

Q WHY DO PEOPLE TEST A BOTTLE BY DRIPPING THE FORMULA ON THEIR WRIST?

A The inside of your wrist is more sensitive than your hand. If the fluid seems hot, it's too hot for your baby to drink. In addition, by turning the bottle over and watching the formula drip out, you can tell if the nipple hole is the right size.

If the formula is dripping out very quickly, the hole is too big and the nipple should be discarded. If there are long pauses between drips or nothing comes out, the hole is too small. It's probably clogged with old formula. Get a new nipple for now. Later you can clear the clog with a clean needle and then wash the nipple with a nipple brush.

Q WHY AM I SUPPOSED TO ALTERNATE SIDES WHEN FORMULA FEEDING?

A Feeding sometimes from the right and other times from the left helps promote balanced visual development. It also helps develop the muscle tone in your baby's neck. If you always feed from the same side, your baby is always looking the same way.

Q WHAT'S SO IMPORTANT ABOUT SKIN-TO-SKIN CONTACT WHILE FEEDING?

A Babies enjoy the closeness of skin-to-skin contact and being able to smell their parent. It helps create a feeling of security. You can cuddle your baby skin-to-skin any time. Feeding is a convenient time because you need to hold your baby close.

When you're giving a bottle, hold your baby in a semi-upright position. That's the best position for bottle-feeding. Never prop a bottle. That could make him choke.

Q HOW MUCH FORMULA DO YOU FEED A BABY?

A The amount depends on your baby's weight and the number of feedings in a twenty-four-hour period. You baby's care provider will tell you how much is best. In the beginning babies usually take about 2 ounces per feeding. However, they don't necessarily take the same amount at each feeding.

When your baby loses interest in the bottle, end the feeding. Discard any leftover formula. Don't coax her to drink what's left. It's important that she recognizes and responds to feelings of fullness. When she's consistently finishing a bottle quickly, add another ounce to that feeding.

AFTERWORD

Somewhere between leaving the birth facility and walking into your living room you may realize the baby in the infant car seat really is yours. This sudden, intense awareness of the thrill and responsibility of being a parent can make you feel like you've just walked a thousand miles. It can be exhausting, even overwhelming. Yet your journey through pregnancy and birth has given you skills and strengths for the road ahead.

Take it easy the first day home. Consider going straight to bed or resting on the couch. It will soon be time for a feeding. Take time to eat. Spend time with your partner, admiring the wonderful addition to your family. Everything else can wait.

Over the next weeks you'll feel stronger and more comfortable taking care of your baby. Having baby stuff everywhere will feel familiar rather than strange. You'll be solidly on the path of parenthood and on a most wondrous journey that will last your lifetime. I wish you the best.

Also from Meadowbrook Press

The Mother of All Baby Name Books
Bruce Lansky, the #1 author of baby name books in North America, has now created *The Mother of All Baby Name Books*. It has over 94,000 baby name choices for prospective parents, complete with origins, meanings, and variations—more information than any other book provides.

Getting Organized for Your New Baby
This interactive book is loaded with practical info and tips on conception, prenatal health, childbirth preparation, baby gear, household management, financial planning, childcare, celebrations, and life with baby. It's newly revised with the latest, greatest knowledge about pregnancy and parenting—plus key facts and resources to help busy parents-to-be make decisions.

Pregnancy, Childbirth, and the Newborn
More complete and up-to-date than any other pregnancy guide, this remarkable book is the "bible" for childbirth educators. It includes a thorough treatment of pregnancy tests, complications, infections, and medications and detailed advice on creating a birth plan.

Eating Expectantly
Dietitian Bridget Swinney offers a practical and tasty approach to prenatal nutrition, combining nutrition guidelines for each trimester with 200 complete menus, 85 tasty recipes, plus cooking and shopping tips. Cited by *Child* magazine as one of the "10 best parenting books of 1993," *Eating Expectantly* is newly revised with the most current nutrition information.

First-Year Baby Care
This is one of the leading baby-care books to guide you through your baby's first year. It contains complete information on the basics of baby care, including bathing, diapering, medical facts, and feeding your baby.

Feed Me! I'm Yours
Parents love this easy-to-use, economical guide to making baby food at home. More than 200 recipes cover everything a parent needs to know about teething foods, nutritious snacks, and quick, pleasing lunches.

**We offer many more titles written to delight, inform, and entertain.
To order books with a credit card or browse our full
selection of titles, visit our website at:**

www.meadowbrookpress.com

or call toll free to place an order, request a free catalog, or ask a question:

1-800-338-2232

Meadowbrook Press • 5451 Smetana Drive • Minnetonka, MN • 55343